Communication & Management Skills for the Pharmacy Technician

Notices

Communication & Management Skills for the Pharmacy Technician

Jody Jacobson Wedret, BPharm, FASHP, FCSHP

Senior Pharmacist
University of California, Irvine Medical Center
Orange, California

Associate Clinical Professor
University of California, Irvine School of Medicine
Irvine, California

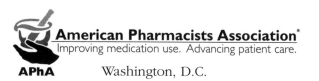

American Pharmacists Association
Improving medication use. Advancing patient care.

APhA   Washington, D.C.

Acquiring Editor: Sandra J. Cannon
Managing Editor: Dean Trackman
Proofreader: Kathleen K. Wolter
Indexer: Mary Coe, Potomac Indexing, LLC
Book Design and Layout: Michele A. Danoff, Graphics by Design
Cover Design: Richard Muringer, APhA Creative Services

© 2009 by the American Pharmacists Association
Published by the American Pharmacists Association
1100 15th Street, NW, Suite 400
Washington, DC 20005-1707
www.pharmacist.com

APhA was founded in 1852 as the American Pharmaceutical Association.

To comment on this book via e-mail, send your message to the publisher at aphabooks@aphanet.org.

Library of Congress Cataloging-in-Publication Data

Wedret, Jody Jacobson.
  Communication & management skills for the pharmacy technician / Jody Jacobson Wedret.
        p. ; cm.
  Includes bibliographical references and index.
  ISBN 978-1-58212-103-1
  1. Pharmacy technicians. I. American Pharmacists Association. II. Title. III. Title: Communication and management skills for the pharmacy technician.
  [DNLM: 1. Pharmacists' Aides. 2. Communication. 3. Pharmaceutical Services--organization & administration. 4. Professional Competence. QV 21.5 W393c 2009]

  RS122.95.W43 2009
  615'.1--dc22
                                        2008052072

How to Order This Book

Online: www.pharmacist.com
By phone: 800-878-0729 (770-280-0085 from outside the United States)
VISA®, MasterCard®, and American Express® cards accepted.

*To Stanley Jacobson and Bob LeWinter,
each of whom in his unique way mentored and inspired me.*

*To my husband, Loren Wedret, without whose
incredible patience, kindness, and support this book
would not have become a reality.*

*A special thanks to Sandy Cannon and
the American Pharmacists Association
for giving me the opportunity.*

Contents

CHAPTER 1
Introduction 1

CHAPTER 2
Communication Skills 5

CHAPTER 3
Customer Service..27

CHAPTER 4
Working with Diverse Patient Populations 47

CHAPTER 5
Professionalism and Ethics in the Workplace................................63

CHAPTER 6
Understanding and Applying HIPAA 87

CHAPTER 7
Role of the Technician in Different Practice Settings....................93

CHAPTER 8
Third-Party Issues 109

CHAPTER 9
Maintaining Medication and Inventory Control Systems 119

CHAPTER 10
Workflow Management...129

CHAPTER 11
Staff Management...145

CHAPTER 12
Team Building, Coaching, and Mentoring 169

CHAPTER 13
Selected Issues Affecting Pharmacy Practice................................179

BIBLIOGRAPHY 195

INDEX 197

CHAPTER | 1

Introduction

A s early as the 1300s, writings mention apothecaries and druggists, as pharmacists were once called. They were proprietors of shops where patients came and described their symptoms. The apothecary listened to the patient, made a recommendation, and compounded the product or products deemed appropriate to treat the condition. Alternatively, physicians made house calls and gave sick patients potions from their black bags.

More recently but still more than a century ago, diagnosing and prescribing began being performed separately by physicians, while pharmacists focused on compounding and furnishing. With the development of pharmaceutical manufacturers in the mid-19th century, the compounding part of the pharmacist's function diminished. As chain drugstores emerged, pharmacists became simply employees rather than proprietors of the operations. Although the traditional drugstore where the proprietor is the pharmacist still exists, more and more community pharmacies are owned and operated by nonpharmacist corporations. During most of this period, hospital pharmacy practice remained primarily a basement operation that was considered an adjunct service.

Even before the role of pharmacists changed, educational requirements for licensure increased. What had once been a profession based on apprenticeship training evolved into one requiring a 3-year, then a 4-year, and eventually a 6-year minimum curriculum for licensure. After 6 years of intense training, graduate pharmacists were disenchanted with the lack of respect and the lack of opportunity 20th-century pharmacy practice offered. They sought a practice model that allowed them to use their specialized knowledge to enhance the outcome of their patients' treatment. The movement that developed to address these concerns was called clinical pharmacy.

Not until the late 1960s and 1970s were hospital pharmacy directors able to acquire space for decentralized pharmacies located throughout hospitals. Working alongside physicians and nurses, pharmacists had the opportunity to be accepted as team members rather than as adjunct service providers. For pharmacists to provide direct patient care again, however, the tasks they had been identified with had to be delegated to others.

Qualified people who could ably assist pharmacists were in demand, but comprehensive on-the-job training for them required time no longer available to pharmacists. Traditionally, in a pharmacist-owned business, the pharmacist's assistant was his wife or an intern/apprentice. In the chain-store practice and in hospital pharmacy, a hired clerk might be trained to do specific tasks. As the notion of delegating frontline responsibilities to nonpharmacists took hold, formal discussions about the need for trained and qualified assistants for pharmacists began. At the urging of pharmacy organizations, state boards of pharmacy developed regulations for the training, role, and registration of technicians.

In many practices today, traditional tasks such as counting, pouring, licking, and sticking are often delegated to technicians. Meanwhile, the role of the pharmacist has evolved to encompass analyzing a patient's condition, reviewing a patient's history, and selecting a therapy to achieve the best outcomes from the treatment options. With pharmacists devoting more time to patient care, the responsibility for managing at least some pharmacy operations will shift to skilled technicians.

CHAPTER 1

In modern pharmacy practices, technicians must be familiar with pharmacy management issues. They need a working knowledge in areas such as customer service, ethics, inventory control, workflow, staffing, and team building. Because their jobs involve a high degree of interaction with colleagues and patients, good communication skills are also essential. It is expected that the frontline people in a pharmacy are welcoming and can solve problems.

This book is intended as both a textbook and a reference handbook to help prepare pharmacy technicians to assume management responsibilities. You will find practical information on the wide range of communication and management issues that come up in pharmacy settings. By exploring the information in the following chapters and working on the activities with colleagues in discussion groups and teams, you will begin to gain the knowledge and hone the skills required to become an effective technician manager.

For More Information

Boussel P, Bonnemain H, Bove FJ. *History of Pharmacy and the Pharmaceutical Industry*. Paris: Asklepios Press; 1982.

Cowen DL, Helfand WH. *Pharmacy: An Illustrated History*. New York: Harry N. Abrams, Inc; 1990.

Posey LM. *Pharmacy: An Introduction to the Profession*. 2nd ed. Washington, DC: American Pharmacists Association; 2009.

Walton SM, Cooksey JA, Knapp KK, et al. Analysis of pharmacist and pharmacist-extender workforce in 1998–2000: assessing predictors and differences across states. *J Am Pharm Assoc*. 2004;44(6):673–83.

CHAPTER | 2

Communication Skills

In all our activities of daily living, we send and receive information. Communication is everything we say and most everything we do. In fact, the primary purpose of a prescription is to communicate. The physician gives the pharmacist information that tells the pharmacist what the physician intends for the patient. Simply stated, communication is the transmission of ideas from the sender to the receiver. The art of communication is best achieved when the sender delivers a message in the fashion best suited for the receiver to comprehend the information and put it to use.

Communication takes the form of verbal conversation, written words, nonverbal motions, and pictures and demonstrations, such as graphs and displays. In this chapter, we will explore several types of communication and focus on the primary forms used in pharmacy practice. Before we look at methods to enhance our ability to communicate effectively, let's look at the different times and places where the various types of communication are used in pharmacy practice.

Conversation, if used well, is one of the most expeditious means of communication because it allows for instant response and verification of the message. During a conversation, we have the ability to ask for immediate feedback. The timeliness of the delivery affords the opportunity to clarify a mistaken idea. Unless recorded, verbal communication allows for statements to be partly rescinded because we can modify or elaborate on our thoughts. Live conversation further allows us to use nonverbal cues as well as words to assess the success of the message and the tone in which it is both delivered and received. The disadvantage of verbal communication is that because of the lack of a permanent record, disagreements about what transpired can only be resolved through mutual agreement.

Written communication has the advantage of providing a record of all that has transpired. In the case of e-mail messages, it also provides a dated history of the communication.

Communication is the transmission of ideas from the sender to the receiver.

Correspondence of any type may be reread, allowing the reader/receiver additional time to understand the message and respond to it. While time delays certainly have the advantage of allowing emotions to subside in a heated issue, the lack of immediate interchange can lead to misunderstandings and misconceptions.

In pharmacy practice, we use verbal and written communication all the time. We answer the phone and greet patients, customers, co-workers, and other health care providers verbally. We provide reports and instructions in writing. We counsel patients verbally and sometimes use charts to help patients understand complex regimens. We receive orders and prescriptions either in writing or verbally. We receive instructions from our supervisors in formal writing, such as policy documents, in informal writing, such as memos and e-mail, or verbally, and updates and shift reports are provided both in writing and verbally.

Another way we communicate among ourselves is through positioning. We often leave information about what needs to be finished by the next shift by placing prescriptions, orders, or other task-related materials in particular prearranged locations. For example, we leave orders or prescriptions that are waiting for the day's delivery in the "hold for drug" area. We leave prescriptions waiting for refill authorization in the "doctor call back" box. We leave medication fill lists on top of patient cassettes, implying that the filled cassettes need to be checked and verified before they are sent to the nursing station. Such a method of organizing the workload by position communicates what needs to be done without words. These positioning practices are established by and for the individual workplace.

Certain conventions have developed over time that make verbal and written communication more productive and less likely to cause confusion or ill will. Let's explore some of these ways that, when used in the right situations, make our communication most effective.

Verbal Communication: In Person

We use verbal communication most of the day. People come in and out of our lives regularly. We greet people in short phrases. We ask for favors. We request help. We give orders. We console. We exchange ideas. We listen to stories and accounts of events. We communicate verbally on the phone and in person. So, if we use this tool all day long, why write about it?

Let's start with the basics. How does verbal communication begin? You initially need to get the attention of the other person. This may be done simply by getting the person on the phone. In person, it might be done by tapping someone on the shoulder. Most often it is done simply by addressing the person by name. Getting the attention of the recipient of the forthcoming message is called engaging.

Why is engaging the person so important? Ask yourself, "Am I really communicating with someone if I ask how she is but then round the next corner before she has even started replying? Is it communication if I talk to someone who knows I'm in the room but who is concentrating on a television program or talking to a patient or a nurse while I talk?"

It is possible to hear without listening. It's a cliché that a husband nods his head and continues to read the paper while his wife engages in "conversation" with him. At the end of the evening, the husband might ask how a particular person is doing only to be informed by his wife that he has already been told about that person. While such a situation makes for a funny scenario on TV, a large part of what makes it funny is that it contains some truth—not only between spouses but also between colleagues. The reality is that many of us tune out speakers. We know that we are being talked to (hearing), but we miss the point (listening).

Listening skills can be improved through active listening. One way to actively listen involves using a pen or pencil and writing down key notes. Another way is to listen for the answers to the what, why, where, when, and how of the message's content:

▌ "What is this person telling me?" focuses on the key points of the message.
▌ "Why is this person telling me this?" makes you stay alert for the importance of the core of the message.

▌ "Where and when am I going to need this?" tells you about the application of the information.

▌ "How am I to use this information?" gives you an understanding of what to do with the information.

Note that while it is helpful to organize the information being received, there is no suggestion that a response be formulated until the whole idea is presented. Doing so while the speaker is still talking often results in miscommunication and misunderstandings.

So, going back to the basic question at the beginning of this section, Why write about verbal communication? It's simple. We need to be aware of the most effective ways to use this powerful tool so that we can get the maximum benefit from it.

Everyone has a different style of communication. For example, some people tend to be long winded in their verbal communication. They tell stories with details and lots of asides in an effort to give the whole picture. Others tend to jump to the point, leaving out details. In business, we accept the different styles of people, but for all of us, it is important to recognize when we need to be succinct. Often, less is more. Sometimes a comment isn't needed at all.

It's often said that two people who live together for a long time can finish each other's sentences. When people work together, they start to learn one another's unspoken language. Responses are often tailored to the person asking the question. For example, the question, "How are we doing?" may elicit different responses depending on who is asking because we use verbal shorthand. Table 2-1 shows a few possible answers to the same question.

TABLE 2-1

Possible Responses to "How Are We Doing?"

Inquirer	Response	What is really being asked?
A colleague passing through	Fine, thanks.	Nothing—it's an informal greeting.
A co-worker	I could use a little help.	How is the project coming?
A lunch buddy	I'll be ready in five minutes.	Are you ready for lunch?
A boss with a deadline	We're almost done.	Is the project completed?

Although the question was simply stated, what it referred to depended on who was asking. This verbal shorthand is fine with people who know each other, but it is important to be clear about your intended message when speaking to people you don't know.

Taking a course in proper conversational English can be helpful in the workplace. Poor grammar and misuse of words can leave a listener confused. Too much slang and the listener can develop a negative opinion of the speaker. The use of nonstandard speech can make a conversation difficult for those who are not native English speakers.

The advantage of verbal communication is that feedback is immediate. You can correct a statement on the spot when you feel that you have been misunderstood. You can get clarification from others while they can still remember the context of their thoughts. Finally, it is quick and relatively effortless and doesn't require supplies.

Body language can convey respect, disdain, pleasure, connection, impatience, and many other unspoken feelings.

Nonverbal Communication

Much of our person-to-person communication is nonverbal. Nonverbal communication is a message transmitted through our body language, personality, and tone of voice. An innocuous message delivered in a huff will be received differently from the same statement made cordially.

Body language can convey respect, disdain, pleasure, connection, impatience, and many other unspoken feelings. Respect is a cultural response. In some cultures, standing when greeting a person of greater importance is considered a sign of respect. In other cultures, it is not necessary. In Mediterranean cultures, both sexes greet each other with big hugs, but in Asian cultures, a handshake may be too forward.

Standing position may also convey messages. Standing too close to someone can be misconstrued as an invasion of the other person's space. It may cause the other person to back away or become distracted. Sometimes, distance sends a message discouraging closeness. Standing over a seated person can be intimidating. Walking backward from a conversation sends a message that the conversation needs to be over.

Seated positions can send messages too. Sitting upright shows that the listener considers the conversation important and is listening. Leaning back in a chair may show that the person is comfortable in the speaker's presence or that he or she is too relaxed and gives the conversation less significance.

It's often said that the eyes are the mirror of the soul. Perhaps this is because many emotions are transmitted through the eyes. In our culture, eye contact is a sign of respect and connection. So looking away during a conversation sends the message that the person is bored, busy, or distracted. A smile shows through the corners of the eyes, making the recipient feel valued and desired. It warms a room and comforts a person not at ease. A furrowed brow shows distrust or disagreement. Rolling of the eyes shows disgust or distrust. What kind of a message do you want potential customers to receive?

Posture isn't the only thing that conveys a message when a person is speaking. Turning away or attending to a chore suggests that the conversation is not interesting or important. Abrupt movements or deliberate actions can be seen as a sign of annoyance. Table 2-2 provides some tips on body language to avoid when you interact with patients.

TABLE 2-2
Body Language to Avoid with Patients

▮ Don't work on another project while talking to a patient.
▮ Don't frown or make faces.
▮ Avoid abrupt turns or sharp movements.
▮ Don't slam down pencils or other items.
▮ Don't show disinterest in the person you are talking with by switching your conversation to other people.

Verbal Communication: Telephone

Bad first impressions are almost impossible to undo. Unless the competing businesses are particularly awful or nonexistent, a bad first impression can cause an irreparable loss of clientele. Often the telephone is the first introduction a customer has to a business. The response a caller receives from the person answering the phone might be the difference between doing business with that operation and going someplace else. For this reason, good telephone etiquette is essential to establishing a friendly, efficient, and businesslike atmosphere.

Nowadays, almost all businesses have automated phone answering systems. A phone tree assists the people *working in the business*—it reduces time spent answering the phone by sorting out calls that may not require immediate attention, and it eliminates the disturbance of staff caused by continually ringing phones. It does, however, put a roadblock in front of the patient trying to reach someone in the pharmacy. Many customers consider it an unnecessary delay.

Good telephone etiquette is essential to establishing a friendly, efficient, and businesslike atmosphere.

Why do people call pharmacies anyway? Patients call pharmacies for store hours, to check the availability of a medication, or to verify that something is ready to be picked up. All these calls are intended to decrease the time spent in the pursuit of the medication. In hospitals, nurses and doctors call for information.

Since phone callers are usually looking to save time, they may be quite frustrated by the time they finally reach the "live" choice on a phone tree. It is important to be helpful and cheerful instead of mirroring a caller's mood. Be responsive, not reactive. It is also important to promptly answer calls from those who opt for a live response. Many pharmacies have a policy that calls should be answered within three rings.

Much research has addressed verbal communication by phone and in person. When a person smiles while speaking, the tone of voice changes significantly. So remember to smile before addressing callers—a pleasant voice helps set the tone for the transaction.

Because patients use the phone to save time, be as efficient as possible. If it is particularly busy, letting callers know that up front saves a lot of stress for them and you. They may wish to call back at a less busy time or have you call them back when you can give them the appropriate level of attention. You can always offer these options.

Before placing someone on hold, always ask if you can do so and wait for an answer. Nothing is more frustrating than calling a pharmacy to see what time it closes (a short response) and being placed on indefinite hold. In addition, by asking to place the caller on hold and waiting for an answer, you may be able to send the call to a more appropriate person.

Sometimes callers are looking for a staff member who is not even working that particular shift. If your co-worker isn't there, ask if you may help. People ask for employees by name because they've had a good experience with that person. Callers may want to ask about pharmacy policy or may need a mailing address or some other information that someone currently working can handle. This approach keeps messages from piling up and gives callers what they need faster than what they expected. Exceeding expectations always makes good business sense. It also shows that the business works as a team.

Before saying good-bye, always ask callers if they need help with anything else. A caller will often have an additional question when prompted. For instance, someone may call to inquire whether a prescription is ready. Suppose it is. You respond that it is and say good-bye. You certainly have provided an appropriate answer to the question, but what if the person also needed to know the cost or the pharmacy hours? Maybe a person is calling from a unit in the hospital to a pharmacy open only part of the day, or a nurse needs the medication and doesn't remember that it is a narcotic and she will need the narcotic log. Asking if you can offer further assistance can expedite the transaction, saving time for both you and the caller. Going the extra mile always makes friends.

Should you be taking a message for a co-worker, make sure you ask for the caller's name and phone number, as well as the reason for the call. While it isn't required that the caller give that information, often the recipient of the message won't recognize the name or won't have the phone number available. By getting the number, you expedite the return call. By determining the nature of the call, you often facilitate the response by allowing the person who will be returning the call time to research an answer if necessary. It also may jog the memory of the person returning the call if the name is unfamiliar.

Auto-attendants and message machines are quite helpful for time management. It is essential, however, that message banks be cleared several times a day. This both frees up space in the limited recording capacity and ensures that the pharmacy staff returns call requests in a timely manner. You can reduce the number of messages by recording key information, such as what time messages are taken off the machine, hours of operation, or when orders or prescriptions can be picked up.

A somewhat rude habit of many executives is having their assistants dial calls. When the recipient of a call is on the phone, the assistant asks the person to hold for the executive. Asking someone to hold for a call you initiated is discourteous. Be as respectful of another's time as you are of your own.

In short, telephones are often used to reduce time spent in pursuit of information. Good business sense necessitates a quick response. Table 2-3 offers some ideas for successfully handling phone calls.

TABLE 2-3
Tips for Successful Phone Calls

- Smile before you say the first words. It changes your voice.
- When you answer a call, introduce yourself and identify the business. This confirms that the caller dialed—or didn't dial—the right number.
- Write down the name of the caller so that you can address the person by name. This shows you are interested in the person and want to be helpful.
- Offer to help if a requested co-worker is not available. Sometimes it is service the caller is after, not just the employee whose name the caller knows.
- Speak into the phone—not to the side of it—so that the caller can hear you.
- Avoid sidebar conversations. Sidebars are conversations in addition to the main conversation you are having on the phone. Engaging in sidebar conversations while you are on the phone is distracting and confusing.
- When you are busy, ask if you may put the caller on hold *and wait for the answer.* The question may be a short one that won't require even the amount of time needed to put the call on hold and return to it.
- Stock notepads and several writing instruments near all phones. This helps you take messages quickly and avoids unnecessary delay when a pen runs dry or a pencil tip breaks.
- Don't place people on hold to demonstrate your importance. Don't make callers wait unnecessarily for you to come to the phone when someone else answers it. This is rude.
- When researching a question for which the answer is not immediately available, ask if the person prefers to wait or be called back. If you know ahead of time that getting the information will take awhile, offer to call the person back. This shows you are respectful of a person's time.

continued on page 14

TABLE 2-3, continued

Tips for Successful Phone Calls

▌ Get the names and numbers for all callers who need to be called back. This will help if they are not where they usually call from or if the information in your database is not current. It also eliminates the step of looking up a number when someone at the pharmacy is ready to return the call.

▌ When it is necessary to transfer a call to another extension, give the complete number to call if the person gets disconnected. If there is someone in particular to speak with after the call has been transferred, also give that name and title. For example, "I'm going to transfer you to our billing department at 456-7890. Ask for Mary, who is our account manager."

▌ When you don't know the best place to refer someone, make a guess at the most reasonable option. Make the call while the other person holds and confirm whether it is the correct department. This prevents the caller from being bounced from one department to another in your business operation.

Written Communication

E-mail

E-mail is a fast way to transmit messages from person to person. It is an impersonal way to send a message to many people in a less time-consuming manner than telephoning or writing each person individually. It is not intended to be used for sending jokes, stories, lengthy dissertations, and other wordy items. This is especially true in a business setting. E-mail at work should be reserved for business use only.

People in important positions may receive several hundred messages a day. Others may receive more than a hundred. Reading through junk mail of any sort is time-consuming. Such mail also ties up computer memory. Understand that memory is computer real estate. The more clutter you have, the more difficult it is for you to move around within the cyberworld. Moreover, sending a lot of unnecessary correspondence increases the potential for viruses to infect your business's software. Viruses can shut down whole systems, resulting in loss of business, lower productivity, and overtime costs to catch up once the problem is solved.

Using e-mail for corresponding on business requests is efficient. It doesn't interrupt the receiver's work. For items that are straightforward, it provides the message most directly and eliminates time spent with pleasantries. E-mail is a quick way to document a request that was made or information that was transmitted.

E-mail does have unique features that, depending on the situation, may or may not be advantageous. First, it removes nonverbal communication, so the mood and tone are difficult to decipher. Second, most e-mail conversations are not carried out in real time, especially in pharmacy operations where much of the day is spent on tasks that are not computer based. The receiver has time to process the message before responding. Third, these conversations are available for replay. They can be forwarded as well. A misunderstanding that can be quickly corrected in verbal communication cannot be as easily corrected via e-mail.

What is good e-mail etiquette? First, the subject line is precise and straightforward. It focuses on the key message, letting the reader know what to expect. Second, the body of the message is concise. If the text of the message is longer than a few paragraphs, it should be attached as a document. Third, the message is organized, and it specifies what needs to be done.

Let's look at some examples of good and inferior e-mail messages.

E-mail should never be answered when you are emotional.

FIGURE 2-1
Brief and Direct E-mail

Example A
Subject: Paper needed

Hi, Jan. Please order two boxes of computer paper for the third-floor satellite. Thanks.

Jess

Example B
Subject: Me again. Guess what?

Hi, Jan. Hope you had a good time at the movie yesterday. I really wanted to see it, but we had other plans. Too bad. Maybe next time. By the way, we need paper. Thanks.

Jess

In Figure 2-1, example A has a short subject line that clearly tells the recipient the purpose of the message. The body of the e-mail is straightforward and simple. There can be no mistake about the request. It will take the recipient little time to read. In example B, the subject line offers no clue about the purpose of the e-mail, and the content is mainly social. The body of the e-mail has so much fluff that a busy recipient might stop reading it—or even delete it—before getting to the key point, which is last. Even then, it omits information about the quantity of paper needed and the location.

When you are writing an e-mail to make a request:

▌ Be concise in your subject line and text.
▌ Remember that less is more.

E-mail should never be answered when you are emotional. If something said in an e-mail message angers you, wait to respond until you are feeling levelheaded. Doing otherwise may cause you problems later.

FIGURE 2-2

Emotional Response in E-mail

Initial e-mail
Subject: Coverage needed this weekend

Hi, everyone.

We need coverage for the following shifts: Saturday am and pm and Sunday pm. Please let me know which shifts you are available to work.

Joan

Response A
Unfortunately, we have plans this weekend. Sorry I can't help out.

Bob

Response B
Good gosh, you're always asking us to work extra. Don't you have any respect for our lives? I guess I can work Saturday morning.

Martin

Imagine that a particular pharmacy has been short-staffed recently because of illness and turnover. The remaining technicians have been repeatedly asked to work overtime, and there is no indication that the end is in sight. Figure 2-2 shows an initial e-mail message from the supervisor and two responses.

Although response A in Figure 2-2 turns down the request, it is clear and to the point. The writer apologizes, expressing some compassion. The employee in response B says he will come in to help, but his message expresses irritation and a degree of anger. The spirit of helping out is missing. Since the response is written, the supervisor can keep it as a record, and it may come back to haunt the employee. When you receive an e-mail that makes you unhappy:

▌ Wait to cool off before responding.
▌ Remember that e-mail messages are conversations that can be saved.

Another potential pitfall with e-mail is the "reply all" feature, which sends an e-mail response to multiple recipients. Limit e-mail responses to those people who need to know. Let's look at the e-mail announcement from a supervisor in Figure 2-3. Assume that it was sent to the entire pharmacy department, which has 75 employees.

By the next day, a flurry of e-mail messages had been sent to the full list. The gist of these messages: "Congratulations,

FIGURE 2-3

Mass-Distribution E-mail

Subject: Staff promotion

Jean Smith has been promoted to head technician. Jean has been a technician in the outpatient pharmacy for the past 4 years. She has received several commendations from the patient thank-you program.

Prior to her experience in outpatient services, Jean worked in the sterile-product area and the neurology satellite. Please join me in wishing Jean good luck in her new position.

Elizabeth

Keep the list of people receiving an e-mail to those who need to be in the loop.

Jean!" Of course, this message doesn't take a lot of time to read, but imagine getting a dozen or more over a two-day period. Every one of the 75 people got many messages that should not have been sent to them.

It's important to keep the list of people receiving an e-mail to those who need to be in the loop. Hit the "reply all" button only when the contents of the e-mail and the corresponding response to it really do apply to all. When you send e-mail messages to a large number of people:

- Make sure your outgoing messages include only those who need to know the information.
- Do the same for your replies.

E-mail messages should be sent only to appropriate recipients. Let's say, for example, that a colleague's husband was hospitalized with a serious ailment. Many people sent cards, flowers, or gifts. Some in the circle visited him in the hospital

FIGURE 2-4

Thank-You E-mail to Colleagues

Subject: John's illness

Dear colleagues:

As many of you know, the last few weeks have been very trying for us. We are very grateful for your outpouring of friendship. Thank you so much for your caring gifts. They have certainly helped us through.

Sincerely,
Mary

FIGURE 2-5

Group Reprimand in E-mail

Subject: Time Cards

All employees need to fill out their own time cards each week by Friday at noon. There are no exceptions. If time cards are not submitted on time, they will not be processed, and paychecks may be held up.

or helped out by making dinner for the family. A week later, the colleague sent the e-mail in Figure 2-4.

The message in Figure 2-4 sounds good, right? So what's wrong? First, some of the recipients did not even know John was ill. Thanking people for something they did not do shows poor organizational skills. It also lacks sincerity. Second, when people take the time to show they care, you should take the time to acknowledge your gratitude individually. The only time group thank-you notes are acceptable is when the gift or assistance is a group effort and the members of the group might not be apparent. When thanking your colleagues:

▌ Be sincere.
▌ Choose your mailing list carefully to avoid embarrassing anyone.
▌ Use personal one-to-one communication when someone has been thoughtful. This includes all gifts.

E-mail should not be used to reprimand a group. The e-mail example in Figure 2-5 was sent to particular staff members by name. This e-mail implies that the people on the list have been negligent in performing a task. What if the information is incorrect and some of the people had not been negligent? Even if everyone in the group was negligent, why should that information be shared publicly? When you have to communicate negative information:

▌ Don't write a group e-mail message if the content may reflect poorly on individuals in the group.
▌ Send it to each person separately.

Table 2-4 summarizes the important do's and don'ts of writing an e-mail message.

TABLE 2-4

E-mail Do's and Don'ts

▌ Do use the subject line to tell the recipient what the e-mail is about.
▌ Do keep the text of the message short and to the point.
▌ Do include everyone if there is an online discussion.
▌ Do attach text documents if the message is going to be long.

continued on page 20

TABLE 2-4, continued
E-mail Do's and Don'ts

▌ Do edit for grammar and punctuation.

▌ Do suggest a conference call instead of e-mail correspondence if the discussion will be long and involved.

▌ Do start a new e-mail when time has elapsed or when you want to discuss a new subject.

▌ Do respond to e-mail requests in a timely manner.

▌ Don't chitchat in e-mail that has business points.

▌ Don't send or answer e-mail when you are emotional.

▌ Don't send e-mail to people who don't need to know.

▌ Don't hit "reply all" if the e-mail is not part of an ongoing discussion.

▌ Don't put negative comments in e-mail.

Leave clear messages about what is needed on items that may carry over to the next shift.

Intradepartmental Notes

It's important to leave clear messages about what is needed on items that may carry over to the next shift or items for which an answer may come back while you are busy with another patient or task. Let's look at the example of orders or prescriptions waiting for clarification. Simply placing a note on an order stating that the doctor will call back leaves the next person who may answer the call without sufficient details to receive the information you need. The omission or the question may not be obvious. Even in a case where a quantity is obviously left off a prescription, it is better to state that information than to have a co-worker guess at what you wanted.

Even a clear message left with the prescriber's office staff doesn't guarantee that the message will be transmitted as clearly to the person returning the phone call. The message may not be completely read or heard by the intended recipient at the prescriber's office. Having complete information allows the receiver of returned calls at the pharmacy to ask additional questions when all the requested information is not given up front. By asking for information, the pharmacy staff member avoids having to make a follow-up phone call, and someone from the prescriber's office does not have to call again should he or she discover that the information given was incomplete. Use abbreviations only if everyone is aware of their meaning. Table 2-5 provides some examples of ambiguous and clear notes.

TABLE 2-5

Examples of Ambiguous and Clear Intradepartmental Notes

Ambiguous	Clear
Verify dose. [Does it mean frequency or quantity?]	How many 5mg tablets per dose? This is an unusual frequency. Verify schedule.
Verify drug.	Patient says this is for anxiety. Verify drug.
MD wcb [Doctor will call back]	MD wcb after 2 pm.
Clarify.	Clarify quantity. Patient says it should be a 2-month prescription.
?	Clarify drug. Handwriting unclear.
Change to formulary med.	Change to med on HealthNet formulary.
Order more.	Order a 2-month supply. Order is for 60. I gave patient 23. Need 37 more. Order the rest and fill remainder. Patient to pick up Thurs.

There are other cases where a lack of information can put the person answering the phone at a great disadvantage. For instance, a phone call to the prescriber for a change of medication may be made on a perfectly written prescription because the profile states that the patient is allergic to the medication or because the insurance company doesn't cover that particular proton-pump inhibitor or sulfonylurea. Without the why, a colleague is left confused and the physician or other prescriber may perceive the call as a waste of time. If there are too many waste-of-time messages to a particular office from your practice site, your phone calls may be less likely to be returned. Therefore, when an immediate answer to an inquiry is not possible, leave a note stating when the call was placed (date and time) and to whom it was placed (prescriber, patient, third party), plus a short description of the reason for the call.

Memos, like e-mail, should be short and to the point.

Memos

Memos, like e-mail, should be short and to the point. Paper memos may be posted for all to read or they can be given to one person. Unlike e-mail, memos directed to individuals are less likely to be forwarded or shared with others. Memos are often used to communicate instructions. Since they may be kept for future reference, the wording has to be clear enough to be read without an explanation.

Today, writers overwhelmingly use the computer to create documents such as memos. Most word-processing programs have spell-check and grammar help, which have made a lot of people lazy in using—and improving—their own skills. One of the problems with spell-check is that it doesn't flag correctly spelled words that are used incorrectly. For instance, when spoken, the sentence "We can meat their after work" sounds the same as the correct sentence "We can meet there after work." Such errors make the writer appear to be uneducated. Yes, spelling and grammar are important.

Letters

Written communication can be read and reread. Since it is usually received without the author present, the receiver can decide when to read it, if at all. Correspondence can be answered at a later date, and an open letter lying around can be read by unintended eyes.

Writing business letters is a little different from writing business memos. Writing formal letters often takes a great deal of time and planning. All forms of writing, however, should display clarity of intent through the use of good English. When a letter is handwritten, good penmanship is essential. Thank-you letters for follow up on interviews or for a job particularly well done are more impressive when personalized by being handwritten. If you cannot write legibly, then it is a good idea to print or type. Remember, the primary purpose of the exchange of all words is to communicate. If the message hasn't been received, communication has not occurred.

Business letters are considered a formal means of business communication. With the possible exception of thank-you notes, letters should always be written in formal style on letterhead or at least with the name and address of the sender as well as of the recipient included. In business writing, the recipient should always be addressed formally (Dr., Mr., Mrs., Ms., not Kathy, Tom, or Dick).

Figure 2-6 (page 24) is a sample letter written to thank a speaker for giving a talk to the local technician group. Another type of business letter asks for information. Some letters confirm a discussion that took place. Figure 2-7 (page 25) is an example that combines both. Table 2-6 provides tips for writing professional business letters.

TABLE 2-6
Business Letter Do's and Don'ts

- Do use formal salutations.
- Do write in clear, complete sentences.
- Do remember to thank people who have been helpful to you.
- Don't use slang.
- Do include your name and address as well as the recipient's address.
- Do clearly state your expectations.
- Do try to limit yourself to one page.
- Don't include unnecessary information that may obscure the main purpose.

Summary

- Communication is an art that includes sending and receiving information.
- In business writing, the purpose should be stated concisely.
- Clarity is important in verbal and written communication.
- Verbal communication allows for a more timely exchange.
- Verbal communication integrates actions with words. Actions include mood, tone of voice, and body language.
- Written communication can be saved, referred to later, and passed around.
- Responding to business situations is best done when a person is past the heat of the moment.

FIGURE 2-6

Business Letter: Thank You

Local Association of Pharmacy Technicians
1301 Pennsylvania Avenue
Washington, DC 20005

June 10, 2008

Jon Deamer, PharmD
Our Little Pharmacy
917 Fenton Street
Silver Spring, Maryland 20910

Dear Dr. Deamer:

Thank you so much for taking the time to speak with our group last Tuesday. Your talk on preventing hypertension gave us some good ideas on how to control our own blood pressure and help our patients as well.

We very much appreciate that you took time out of your busy schedule to talk with our group. The feedback on your talk was very good. We hope you'll consider talking to us again in the near future.

Sincerely,

Julie Ruth
Secretary

FIGURE 2-7

Business Letter: Information

ABD Pharmacy
101 Broad Street
Alexandria, Virginia 22314

July 31, 2008

Mr. Donald Travers
Jackson Pharmaceutical Supply Company
3 Jackson Tower
Chicago, Illinois 60625

Dear Mr. Travers:

This letter is to confirm receipt of the six boxes of midazolam
1mg/ml that you sent last Wednesday. We appreciate the
speed with which you got that to us.

We will need an additional six boxes early next week to
allow surgeries to proceed as scheduled. Please let us know
when you ship them.

I understand that your shortage will be over soon. I'm
wondering when we may expect the midazolam 5mg/ml
strength.

Sincerely,

Donna Parker
Lead Technician

ACTIVITIES

1. Divide into groups and role play using pharmacy scenarios.

2. Save the subject lines and text of e-mail messages you've received. Analyze them for clarity and appropriateness.

For More Information

Berger BA. *Communication Skills for Pharmacists: Building Relationships, Improving Patient Care.* 3rd ed. Washington, DC: American Pharmacists Association; 2009.

Morrison EK. Communication. Chap. 7 in *Leadership Skills: Developing Volunteers for Organizational Success.* Cambridge, Mass: Da Capo Press; 1994.

Nygaard LC, Queen JS. Communicating emotion: linking affective prosody and word meaning. *J Exp Psychol Hum Percept Perform.* 2008;34(4):1017–30.

Sigband NB. *Effective Communication for Pharmacists and Other Health Care Professionals.* Upland, Calif: Counterpoint Publications; 1995.

CHAPTER | 3

Customer Service

Most people would not place a visit to the pharmacy high on a list of things they really want to do. Those who go to a pharmacy are often sick or are closely involved with people who are. It is a necessary annoyance that usually costs them more than they wish, even if they have good insurance and a minimal co-pay. While few ever suggest that the price of their specialty coffee is excessive, pharmacy costs seem to be everyone's pet gripe. And besides that, browsing at a pharmacy is not as exciting as it is at a car dealership, an electronics store, a high-end fashion store, or a jewelry store.

Before we start talking about customer service, we have to understand what kind of service we provide. For the most part, pharmacy practice includes consultative services for patients and providers, medication management services, and medication delivery. Traditionally, even though consultation was a part of the practice, pharmacy health care delivery was product driven. While delivery of medications and durable medical equipment is still part of many practices, the field has evolved so that compensated service and consultation are key components of what is offered in most settings. Service may include monitoring medication outcomes, coaching patients to help them succeed with their personalized regimens, or adjusting doses to ensure or control drug responses.

What Can We Do to Attract and Keep Patients and Customers?

Those traditionally thought of as customers in pharmacy practice are patients. But anyone we come in contact with should also be treated as customers. Such people may include other health care professionals asking for advice, insurance company personnel who may want to set up a contract for pharmaceutical services for their insured population, and even the people picking up prescriptions for patients.

The key word in good customer service is respect.

In any business, new customers can be attracted by advertising. In a service-oriented field, retaining clientele is accomplished by building relationships. Building relationships involves everyone working in the pharmacy. Because the technician is often the first face that patients and customers encounter in the pharmacy, the technician's interaction with them can significantly influence the success of the business.

The key word in good customer service is respect. The consummate health professional respects the fact that people differ in many ways—for example, in beliefs, opinions, culture, religion, appearance, and education. It is not necessary to agree with people to respect them. Respect means treating people with the same care that you would if they were your loved ones and valuing them simply because they are human beings. We will also explore many ways to communicate respect in the following chapters.

Basic Business Reception

Imagine walking up to the pharmacy to drop off a prescription and seeing only the top of the technician's head at counter level. The technician is sitting on a box and talking on the phone. It becomes apparent that the conversation is personal. You wait a few minutes. Realizing that you have not been noticed and certainly not acknowledged, you clear your throat in an attempt to make your presence known. The technician glares up at you and then returns to the phone conversation. Several minutes later, he hangs up, gets up, and seeing your prescription in hand, greets you by saying, "Is this all you want?" Consider how a nurse from a busy unit might react to such an encounter when visiting a hospital pharmacy.

Let's consider the correct way to receive clients at a business. Greeting any client with a smile goes a long way toward establishing goodwill, which you may need should you not be immediately able to deliver what the person wants. After being welcomed with a smile, a hello, and the friendly words, "How may I help you?" even the most stressed customer relaxes a little. Should a wait be necessary to allow you sufficient time to deliver the request or item, you are more likely to get approval with a professional greeting than if it appears to the customer that you are biding time until your shift is over. In other words, the perception may not be accurate, but it is always real to the beholder. If the operation is perceived to be lax and casual, then customers for whom accuracy and efficiency are positive attributes for a professional will not be putting their trust in the company or giving it their business.

Attributes for Successful Professional Communication

To help others, you need to be compassionate, sympathetic, empathetic, sincere, and encouraging, depending on the situation.

Compassion

Compassion allows us to actively seek to ease the pain or suffering of another. In health care, this is usually accomplished through problem solving and the delivery of services. Such a service might be timely filling and dispensing of medication. At other times, it includes offering a solution to a problem the patient is struggling with.

How is compassion expressed in a pharmacy situation? One example is acknowledging that a patient may be uncomfortable standing and offering a chair. In another situation, the pharmacist might give a patient a dose of the prescription to take while the technician is preparing the prescription so that the patient can benefit from the medication as soon as possible. Or, a harried mother might be distraught because she has a sick child waiting to be picked up from school and also needs a prescription filled for the child. The technician might suggest that she leave the prescription, pick up the child, and return for the medication. People experiencing stressful situations may not be able to solve their problems rationally.

In the inpatient setting, compassion might mean delivering a medication to the nurse who is harried and unable to leave the nursing unit to come to the pharmacy, even if that is not normal procedure. Sometimes, taking an extra minute to listen to someone vent is the compassionate thing to do whether or not you are in a hurry. Compassion can be summed up as treating others as people, not as task units.

Sympathy and Empathy

Sympathy is the experience of similar emotions, and empathy allows us to understand and acknowledge emotions without actually experiencing them. Without being sick ourselves, we can understand and appreciate how being sick may make a person frustrated, unhappy, uncomfortable, impatient, or crotchety. This understanding allows us to forgive behavior we might otherwise find offensive and to carry on with fulfilling our health care mission of providing good pharmaceutical care to all our patients, including those with bad attitudes.

Sympathy and empathy also help us recognize how another might want to be treated because we can imagine how we would want to be treated in the same situation. They allow us to project ourselves into a situation so that we can genuinely be there for others.

Sincerity

Going through the mechanics of good service is not enough. Think about the expression "Actions speak louder than words." A colleague relayed the following story demonstrating this concept.

The colleague observed a patient consultation done by a pharmacy intern who was particularly well prepared. The intern introduced herself, said all the right words, and made all the key points during the consultation portion of the interview, but she never gained the patient's respect. It was not because the intern should have been even more articulate. It wasn't that she got flustered and quit. It wasn't even because the intern left out key information, because she did not. The intern failed the task because she *failed to listen* to the patient, and in failing to listen, she failed to demonstrate sincerity and commitment to the patient. During the consultation, the intern addressed the patient by name three times. Each time the intern mispronounced the patient's name, and each time the patient corrected her. All three times, the patient was ignored. The intern was so absorbed in what she wanted to say and how she said it that she did not converse with the patient. Instead, she talked *at,* not *to,* the patient. Failing to acknowledge the patient's correct name was perceived as a serious sign of disrespect. It certainly mattered to the patient, since the patient repeatedly corrected the intern.

To deal with a name that is hard to pronounce, you can apologize and offer to try the best you can. You can request that the person say the name more slowly or repeat it. Sometimes, it is helpful to ask the person to break it down into syllables, spell it, or give you another word that sounds like it. It is also helpful to repeat the name just after you are corrected. This reinforces how to pronounce it. The repetition also gives the person another opportunity to correct you. Even if you aren't able to catch on, the fact that you attempted to get it right will be perceived as caring.

Part of patient care is helping patients progress with their treatment plans even if they experience a setback.

Encouragement

Part of patient care is helping patients progress with their treatment plans even if they experience a setback. Encouragement is the ability to motivate people to proceed in a direction even when they get disheartened and want to stop.

When you encourage, you need to do it sincerely and with perspective. A person who runs five miles a day should understand that a patient's accomplishment of walking around the block may not seem like a lot by comparison, but to a person who was completely inactive before, once around the block *is* a big deal. A young adult who lost 10 pounds in a week to fit into a prom dress may not realize how difficult it was for a patient to lose 1 pound in 2 weeks. As health care providers and workers, we need to realize that it may be through small steps that our patients approach their goals. The sense of accomplishment and motivation derived from a simple observation such as, "You look like you've lost weight," or, "You're looking athletic today," can be the perfect motivator for a person who is losing initiative or hitting a weight-loss plateau. It also invites discussion of what worked or what may be the next step needed to continue progress. In other words, it isn't necessary to wait until a 250-pound person has reached the goal weight of 120 pounds before noticing.

Winning in Business Is Not the Same as Winning a Debate

Have you ever heard someone describe another person as rude and thought that the person being described wasn't rude at all? Have you ever been someplace where it seemed as if the employees couldn't be any slower and the people you

ACTIVITY

Let's look at the case of a long-term patient at a particular pharmacy.

Mrs. Saunders is 52 years old and was recently diagnosed with diabetes. She is overweight. She has two sons who are in their early twenties, and she lives alone.

The doctor ordered Mrs. Saunders to check her blood glucose four times a day and return to the clinic in 2 weeks. She came to the pharmacy for the blood glucose monitoring kit and supplies. The pharmacist instructed her on how to monitor her sugar with the kit. The doctor's office called 2 weeks later to ask if the kit could be replaced because the patient said it didn't work. Two weeks later, the same thing occurred, although there had been no problems with the many other blood glucose monitoring kits that had been sold recently.

At this point, the pharmacist asked the patient to demonstrate how she monitored her blood glucose. The patient responded, "I don't like to prick my finger."

▌ **How can the pharmacist respond to the patient? Write down or discuss several responses that show compassion, sympathy, empathy, sincerity, or encouragement and that will motivate the patient. After you have come up with your responses, continue reading about this case. For the sentences in italics, identify the attributes the pharmacist is using in her interactions with the patient.**

By asking the patient to demonstrate how she used the monitoring device, the pharmacist discovered the problem. The pharmacist was able to determine that the problem lay with the patient, not the device.

First, the pharmacist acknowledged that nobody likes pricking a finger. She also noted that checking blood glucose can be cumbersome and time consuming.

The pharmacist patiently explained what could happen in uncontrolled diabetes. Because the patient hoped to see her sons married and to play with grandchildren, the pharmacist had a relatively easy time showing the advantages of monitoring blood glucose. The pharmacist described how uncontrolled diabetes can lead to foot infections and complications that frequently result in amputation. *With proper monitoring, the patient would be able to walk down the aisle at her sons' weddings instead of having to use a wheelchair.* The pharmacist also explained that loss of vision is often a consequence of uncontrolled blood sugar. *If she gained control of her diabetes and kept her blood sugar under control, she would increase her chances of actually seeing her grandchildren.* By putting the risks into a value system that coincided with the patient's, the pharmacist was able to motivate her.

Since the patient was a regular at the pharmacy, the staff and pharmacist had many opportunities to see her. *Each time, they asked how her diabetes was doing.*

Over time, the patient shared her progress and news of her family with the pharmacy staff. At one time, she told the staff that the doctor wanted her to "eat better and exercise more."

▌ **What suggestions can you make that offer the patient specific ideas on how to accomplish this?**

Several years later, one of the patient's sons died. Mrs. Saunders said that she hadn't felt like living since she lost her son. She had stopped monitoring her blood glucose even though she was now down to monitoring just two days a week.

▌ **How should the pharmacy staff respond to this news?**

Of course, the staff extended their sympathy. They helped her see that she still had one son to live for and helped her get back to her exercise routine. The last time the patient visited the pharmacy, she was still doing well.

Notice how different situations in the patient's life offered the staff a variety of opportunities to show compassion, sympathy, empathy, and encouragement in sincere ways that helped the patient achieve optimal health.

were with said that the employees were quicker than usual? It's an old saying that one person's paradise is another's hell. This is what perception is about, and perception is the truth to the person beholding it.

There are certain universal signs of good service, yet there will always be someone who feels wronged. Perception is how customers feel they are being treated by the staff. Reality is what is actually occurring. Reality is based on facts. Feelings are based on subjective and nondebatable factors that may be accumulated from experience and background. It's important to try to please as many customers as possible while realizing that no one can be all things to all people.

Let's think about the following situation. An angry patient approaches the pharmacy and says, "How long are you going to make me wait today?" The technician could answer in several ways. Let's see how each of these answers might be perceived.

Scenario 1

Patient: How long are you going to make me wait today?

Technician: We don't make you wait.

Patient (interrupting): Sure you do. It always takes so long here.

Technician: No it doesn't. Besides, you can go next door for ice cream or go home and do something else for a while. You choose to wait.

Note that the technician can be perceived as argumentative in the first response, probably only making the customer angrier. The second response is confrontational even if it is correct. Now let's look at another way to address this patient.

Scenario 2

Patient: How long are you going to make me wait today?

Technician: Just as soon as I get some information from you, we'll get right on it. Have you been to our pharmacy before?

The technician immediately gets down to business. Many patients will be satisfied that the technician is taking care of them, but some will still press for an answer.

Patient: Yes, but it's been awhile. By the way, I moved. The new address is 123 North Main. Anyway, I don't have much time. How long are you going to make me wait?

Technician: It'll be about 20 minutes. We have several people before you. Would you like us to take care of this while you take care of other things and come back later? We close at 5 o'clock.

This approach acknowledges that the patient may have other things to do and offers alternatives to waiting.

Scenario 3
Humor is another approach to managing the situation. This reply assumes that you know the patient fairly well or that you are good at delivering these kinds of lines. It should be used only with those you know will not be offended.

Patient: How long are you going to make me wait today?

Technician: I don't know. How long have you got?

Scenario 4
When dealing with people who believe that the service is bad, you should ask enough questions to determine what they feel the problem is. Their "truth" or perception is what counts. Sometimes, a comment made while searching for the real issue can help you turn around something and enhance your operation. Let's look at another approach.

Patient: How long are you going to make me wait today?

Technician: You sound upset. Right now, our wait is about 15 to 20 minutes.

Patient: Well, you're the first honest one. They always tell me it will be 5 minutes, and it always takes forever. You would think I had nothing better to do than stand around waiting for you people.

In the last statement, the patient has told us she feels deceived ("You're the first honest one"). She has told us that the wait is underestimated. (We know it doesn't really take forever, but debating that is not helpful to anyone.) She doesn't feel valued by the pharmacy ("You would think I had nothing better to do"). While this patient's retort may sound negative and even condescending, by actively listening, we are able to appreciate the patient's real issues.

This patient has given us feedback that we should use as a measure to evaluate our effectiveness in communicating.

Perhaps we routinely say 5 minutes without thinking about it or finding out how long it really takes. The patient has also let us know that we may not be engaging our patients to the point that they feel valued. Finally, we have conveyed no sincerity, respect, or sympathy and empathy, instead treating the patient like a number.

The take-home message from these scenarios: take care of the patient. By engaging in active listening, we can improve the situation and address a patient's concerns. Instead of getting into a debate on the merits of a complaint, focus on righting the wrong. You win if you retain the patient, come out even if you prevent the patient from spreading bad stories about your business or you, and lose only if the patient leaves the business upset and is determined not to come back and to make sure that nobody else does either.

Handling Patients of Different Ages

The people who visit a pharmacy vary in age. Infants through adolescents are usually accompanied by a parent or parents. While it is respectful to address the adults, it is good patient care to include children if they are old enough to participate in the conversation. How much of the conversation you direct toward children and how you address them depends on their age, maturity, and interest level. Even older preschoolers know their names and addresses. By allowing them to give it to you rather than addressing all questions to the adults, you will make children feel important. Building self-respect and giving children attention is not only good business, it also makes for better-behaved children in your business. Obviously, if a child is shy and you are busy, then the adult can expedite the exchange of information.

Regardless of age, adults are best addressed by title and last name until it is clear that a more familiar address is welcomed. It is better to be considered overly respectful than rude and ill-mannered. Of course, if the patient or customer is someone you and your family have dinner with regularly and your children play with each other, such formality would be deemed unnecessary in most communities. For strangers or people you aren't acquainted with, first names should be reserved until a genuine relationship has been established. Some regions of the country are likely to be more formal than others, so the time frame necessary for considering familiarity established may vary. Of course, if someone requests that you use his or her given name, then it is appropriate no matter how long you have known each other.

In contrast, children should be addressed by first name. Inviting them to be part of the conversation makes them feel important. For children with chronic or severe ailments, the added bit of respect helps ease fears that they are sick because they did something wrong or are unworthy of good health. Children of preschool through school age are most prone to these kinds of feelings. For adolescents, contracting an illness at the age when they are first developing their sense of self and trying to fit in can be devastating. If you can make a young patient feel respected and important or grown up, you can make a big difference in that person's development of self-respect. You also are likely to make a big difference in that patient's adherence to the medication regimen. Remember, making the patient part of the process increases the success of the treatment plan.

Making the patient part of the process increases the success of the treatment plan.

Today, many more people are living longer. For a number of the elderly, aging is accompanied by dementia from different causes. Nonetheless, not everyone suffers from dementia, although reaction time often is slower. Because of failing health, many lose their independence and come to rely on their children or younger neighbors. Realizing that they are not as sharp as they once were and need to rely on others can make older people feel like children and cause depression. While it may be more efficient to get information from younger people, it is polite and helps endorse worthiness to wait for elderly patients to interact with you if they are capable.

Being mindful of patients' abilities boils down to being respectful. How you handle various situations is a measure of compassion, empathy, and sincerity. Illness can be frightening for many people. It can be depressing because it confirms their frailties and mortality. It's our job as health care providers and adjunct personnel to be aware of patients' emotions and to support patients. Respect helps build people up.

Imagine that you are older and because of your infirmity must wait for your adult child to make time for you. Except for a once-a-week outing, you are homebound and isolated. Two out of 4 weeks, your day out involves a trip to the pharmacy. For some of those outings, you need to deal with

The goal of problem solving when you are dealing with an unhappy patient is to create a win-win solution.

your adult child's impatience. You may be aware that the trip to the pharmacy is causing your grandchild to miss part of a birthday party. How would your demeanor be different with these three greetings?

▪ "Yes?"
▪ "Hello, how can I help you?"
▪ (With a smile) "Hello, Mrs. Turner. How are you doing today? Have you baked anything new lately?"

The first greeting is impersonal. While it acknowledges that the person is in front of the technician, it is perfunctory. Such a greeting can accomplish the business at hand, but it neither invites nor helps create a lasting relationship. The second greeting is unimaginative and impersonal but a little friendlier. It superficially establishes a relationship and certainly leaves the door to one open.

The last greeting confirms that you have a relationship with Mrs. Turner. Name recognition makes people feel important. Knowing something about her hobbies or interests adds sincerity to the interaction. Such a greeting will go a long way toward making Mrs. Turner's day. It confirms her worthiness to her helper/child. With someone you haven't seen before, a warm, smiling hello and even a superficial question about anything will help personalize the interaction because it invites discovery and a relationship.

Dealing with Difficult Patients

It has been said, "The customer is not always right. However, the customer is always the customer." Acting in a professional manner does not mean that you have to admit to being wrong when you are right. It does mean that you have to make the situation as right as reasonably possible in the patient's eyes. While there are some patients who enjoy the fight and will never find things good enough, it is wise to adopt a policy of thinking that all people are reasonable until proved otherwise and that their requests are also reasonable. The goal of problem solving when you are dealing with an unhappy patient is to create a win-win solution—the patient goes away happy and returns for the next pharmacy need. This does not have to mean "giving away the store."

Asking for the patient's input into the resolution of a problem encourages the patient to be part of the process and to buy in to the resolution. You do not have to sell the idea as a good one.

Sometimes you can redirect a patient who is difficult. This method is used by parents in controlling the behavior of small children, but it can also be quite effective with adults who are difficult. Let's go back to that opening line from the unhappy patient:

Patient: How long are you going to make me wait today?

Technician: If you can just give me your address and answer a few questions, we'll be able to start right away.

In this example, the technician redirects the patient's attention from a confrontation to the resolution.

The LAST Approach

There are many methods to calm angry patients or customers. We've explored a few. Let's look at one in particular—LAST—that incorporates many of the ideas we've discussed. LAST stands for listen, acknowledge, solve, thank. This technique can also be used to solve interpersonal issues between co-workers, nonpatient customers, and patients.

The first step is to *listen*—allowing patients to tell their side of the issue. While you may or may not agree with a patient's assessment of the situation, actively listening goes a long way toward helping you solve the problem. Active listening involves making a good effort to hear everything the patient has to say and, if in person, watching body language as well. It also involves separating the tone from the message. Trying to formulate your response while listening to the speaker often results in a response that has nothing to do with the real problem. You want to hear every word because often the problem stated initially isn't the problem at all.

As we look at the following conversation, let's assume that the pharmacy is particularly busy, and three waiting prescriptions are ahead of this patient.

Technician: Good afternoon. May I help you?

Patient: I don't know. You people always take so long. I'm just trying to get my prescription filled, and it seems like it's taking all day. First I spent 2 hours at the doctor's office. Then it took 45 minutes to get here. How much longer do I have to wait? Is this going to take forever?

Without active listening, the technician might have stopped listening after the accusation that the pharmacy always takes more time than the patient feels is necessary. The technician might have gotten defensive and reacted by informing the patient that the pharmacy takes the right amount of time or that it takes no longer than any other pharmacy to fill a prescription. However, if we review the entirety of the patient's comments, it is clear that the patient is frustrated by spending much of the day pursuing medical care, *including* the prescription.

What is a good response? Consider the following:

1. "We can only work so fast. There are three people in front of you. We'll get yours out as soon as possible."
2. "If you don't like the way we do business, why do you keep coming here?"
3. "You don't have to be insulting. We're doing the best we can."
4. "I can see that you are frustrated by the long waits you've had all day. We'll try to get you out of here as soon as possible. Why don't you have a seat, and I'll get started on your prescription?"
5. "Sounds like you've had a tough day. Would you like to leave the prescription and come back later for it? I can call you when it's ready."

The first response is clearly straightforward and to the point. It reacts to the patient's comment about the speed at which the pharmacy team works. It gives the patient the information about the length of the wait. But it fails to acknowledge the patient's frustration. Response 2 is clearly argumentative. While the technician may feel that way, it is not good business practice to confront emotion with emotion. Response 3 is defensive. In health care, it is not about you. The patient is the most important person.

Depersonalizing attacks on the pharmacy is the best plan. Both 4 and 5 acknowledge the patient's mood in an empathetic manner and offer a reassuring solution without inconveniencing other patients. While comforting the patient by acknowledging his or her frustration, the technician has zeroed in on the key issue. This avoids confrontation and a long conversation.

By acknowledging people's feelings, you make them feel heard and important.

The *A* in LAST stands for *acknowledge*. By acknowledging people's feelings, you make them feel heard and important. In responses 4 and 5 above, notice that the technician has not said the patient is right to feel that way. It is not your position to judge the appropriateness of a mood or feeling. It is your job to provide good pharmaceutical care and make your patients and customers feel valued and important. By acknowledging the aggravation a patient has endured, you give support and validate that you have listened and heard the person.

The *S* in LAST stands for *solve*. Let's look at another scenario for customer service. This incident took place at an airport before 9/11, when security was less tight than it is today. Note how supremely well orchestrated this turnaround by the service provider is.

An airline ran frequent shuttles between two cities roughly 500 miles apart (one hour flying time). The 4 o'clock flight was canceled. A passenger arrived for the 4 o'clock flight at about 2:45 pm and noticed that it had been canceled; the two remaining choices were the 3 o'clock flight and the 5 o'clock flight. The passenger sprinted 500 yards and made it to the gate of the 3 o'clock flight with 5 minutes to spare.

Passenger: I see you canceled the 4 o'clock flight 2 hours ago. Don't you people have any respect for our time? When exactly were you going to tell me?

Customer service representative: Even more important, can I get you on this flight?

Imagine what would have happened if the customer service representative had gotten into a discussion about informing customers and the airline's policy. Most likely there would have been a verbal fight. Possibly a manager would have been called, which might have gotten the passenger a

Adopting the mind-set of solving the real issue goes a long way toward pleasing the customer and avoiding conflict.

free ticket. But look at the passenger's complaint: "Don't you people have any respect for our time?" Time is the passenger's concern. The passenger does not say, "With the amount of money I spend with the airline, you should..." Instead, the complaint points directly to the issue of time. Focusing on getting the passenger home early solved the passenger's time issue. It was a win-win solution. Pursuing a discussion on the responsibility of informing all passengers of delayed or canceled flights likely would have resulted in the passenger missing the first flight and the creation of a disgruntled customer for the airline—a lose-lose situation.

Now let's adapt this type of problem solving to a pharmacy situation. In the outpatient setting, suppose the pharmacy is unable to fill a prescription because the medication was not delivered. A patient rushes in at the end of the day. When the technician tells the patient that the prescription is not ready, the patient responds, "When were you going to tell me? You people are so incompetent." Instead of defending the pharmacy, suppose the technician responds, "Even more important, how fast can I get the medication for you?"

A typical situation in an inpatient setting is a nurse calling the pharmacy to request a medication that the technician knows has either been sent or delivered in the patient's cassettes.

Nurse: You forgot to send the noon dose of metoclopramide for Mrs. Jones.

Technician: No we didn't. It's in the cassette. I filled it myself.

The technician may be right. He may even have had a previous experience of running over to the nursing station and finding the medication. This nurse may be particularly exasperating—someone who routinely cannot find medication. Nonetheless, should the technician make the patient suffer for the nurse's incompetence? The answer is no. The most important objective is getting the medication to the patient, so the technician is ultimately going to end up providing a new dose. It is not necessary to get into a discussion over who is right. Adopting the mind-set of solving the real issue goes a long way toward pleasing the customer and avoiding conflict.

In some cases, getting to the bottom line, as demonstrated in the previous examples, is not the practical solution. Suppose you have a patient who accuses the pharmacy of shorting him one to five units of medication each time. The first several times the pharmacy decides to make good without question. After awhile, though, it becomes evident that this is the way the patient stretches his prescription dollar. In this type of case, problem solving has to take on a new dimension. The pharmacist may instruct you to count the tablets or capsules in front of the patient and have the patient sign off on it to verify the correct amount was given. Of course, you shouldn't say, "We're going to count this out with you because you are always making false accusations and we're tired of it." Instead, you might suggest, "Why don't we count this together so that we're sure you get the right amount this time?"

Solving problems may take some creativity. Your colleagues may offer ideas that you had not considered. Sometimes you'll get simple complaints, such as, "You're always so busy when I come in." To this patient, you might suggest coming in during specific times when you are usually less busy. Sometimes a physician will call and say that it is always difficult to get a live person on the line. For such customers, you might provide another line with a direct number. Sometimes the solution to a problem involves suggesting dosage forms that the patient or prescriber did not know were available or offering less expensive alternatives to what was prescribed. While giving this kind of advice is truly in the pharmacist's domain, being familiar with the classes of drugs and the formularies of the common insurance plans makes you an asset to the pharmacist.

Finally, the *T* in LAST stands for *thank you*. Whether or not you agree that the problem is a system problem rather than a patient-specific problem, you still should be grateful that it has been brought to your attention. In this context, a system problem is one where the outcome is a result of how you do business. A patient-specific problem is one that only affects that patient or similar patients. Why should you be grateful to hear about problems? First, it is helpful to have people give you feedback. If you truly believe in performance improvement, then both positive and negative feedback are necessary to fully evaluate the systems that are in place. Second, you should appreciate people who take the time to complain rather than simply leave your business without giving you the opportunity to correct issues. Finally, thanking people makes them feel appreciated and valued. It can warm even a tepid heart and frequently is enough to make the patient or customer want to give the pharmacy a second chance.

LAST works if there is an issue to resolve. Sometimes a person may be in a bad mood and there is nothing the pharmacy did wrong. Confronting the mood directly if you have time to listen may be the best approach. For instance, you notice that a nurse is being particularly curt. This is evident from his failure to greet you and also from his body language. Stating the obvious—"You seem a bit on edge this morning"—may open up a discussion on how he had a fight with his wife or how he was late getting the kids to school and forgot their lunches. The statement shows concern on your part and gives the other person an opportunity to vent. The nurse's realization that the behavior is noticeable and your willingness to listen may be enough to turn his mood around and make the rest of the day go better for everyone. It establishes you—and the pharmacy—as caring and concerned. What a great reputation!

Summary

Customer service involves more than handing over what the patient or customer came for. Treating everyone respectfully ensures a satisfied clientele and return business. Connecting with a patient or customer through compassion, sympathy, empathy, sincerity, and encouragement often helps develop the relationship necessary to provide service tailored to the person's needs. Problems are bound to come up, and one useful method for solving them is LAST: listen to the person's perspective on the issue; acknowledge the person's feelings; solve the problem, focusing on a win-win result; and thank the person for bringing the problem to your attention.

For More Information

Curtiss FR, Fry RN, Avey SG. Framework for pharmacy services quality improvement—a bridge to cross the quality chasm. Part I. The opportunity and the tool. *J Manag Care Pharm.* 2004;10(1):60–78.

Desselle SP, Zgarrick DP. *Pharmacy Management: Essentials for All Practice Settings.* 2nd ed. New York: McGraw-Hill Medical; 2008.

Gulati R. Silo busting: how to execute on the promise of customer focus. *Harvard Bus Rev.* 2007;85(5):98–108.

Gulati R, Oldroyd JB. The quest for customer focus. *Harvard Bus Rev.* 2005;83(4):92–101,133.

Levin RP. Developing lifetime relationships with patients: strategies to improve patient care and build your practice. *J Contemp Dent Pract.* 2008; 9(1):105–12.

Miller SR. Scrip for success: Kentucky family practice uses electronic prescription to improve efficiency, revenue and customer service. *Health Manag Technol.* 2003; 24(10):20–1.

Nau DP, Chi C, Mallya U, et al. Member satisfaction related to self-reported cost share and difficulty in obtaining prescription drugs in a university pharmacy benefit plan. *J Manag Care Pharm.* 2007;13(2):135–41.

Slowiak JM, Huitema BE, Dickinson AM. Reducing waiting time in a hospital pharmacy to promote customer service. *Qual Manag Health Care.* 2008;17(2):112–27.

Tomczyk DJ. Improving managed care value through customer service. *Healthc Financ Manage.* 2002;56(6):38–42.

CHAPTER | 4

Working with Diverse Patient Populations

The United States is a diverse nation that has absorbed an array of cultures over its history. People have emigrated from countries across the globe, bringing their beliefs and traditions with them. While these cultures have become part of the fabric of American life, individuals express them in different ways and to varying degrees.

As health care providers, we encounter this diversity one patient at a time. A lack of knowledge about the customs and expectations of other cultures can result in misunderstanding, inadvertent insults, and, subsequently, a loss of business. Thus, it is important to develop an awareness of other cultures and belief systems.

What is meant by culture? Culture can be defined as "the sum total of ways of living built up by a group of human beings and transmitted from one generation to another."[1] We often think of culture as a group's expression of its principles through various forms, including dance, visual arts, theater, architecture, sports, meal habits, and dress.

TABLE 4-1
Important Cultural Influences on Health Care

Life-Cycle Events with Cultural Variations	Health Issues with Cultural Variations	Social Issues with Cultural Variations
Birth	Caregiver-physician vs. faith healer	Family hierarchy
Adulthood	Western medication vs. herbal remedies	Communication styles
Marriage	Science of medicine vs. religion or spirituality	Faiths and religion
Death	The patient as decision maker vs. decision maker for the patient	

Certainly, studying these forms of expression can help us gain an understanding of a particular culture. The basis of this outward display of culture, however, is the group's philosophy, ethical makeup, customs of interaction between people, and rules of personal conduct.

Every culture deals differently with major life-cycle events, as well as with the concepts of health and illness. Table 4-1 lists cultural influences that may affect patients' comfort or explain their approach to health care. So, what does this have to do with pharmacy practice?

Cultural Competence

Cultural competence defines how you use compassion, sympathy, empathy, and encouragement in a manner tailored to the specific patient. By becoming familiar with the norms of other cultures, you are prepared to handle common situations that arise with patients whose backgrounds are different from your own and who expect resolutions different from those most familiar to you. While it is not required to change all your actions to fit into the norms of all others, being able to adapt to a patient's cultural norm may ease a tense situation or build a bridge to a patient for life. Developing cultural competence by acquiring a knowledge base will allow you to adapt practices within reason to make people most comfortable in the pharmacy environment.

The rituals of a culture are often more ingrained in elderly people, but younger people may also hold their cultural norms in high esteem. Sometimes members of the younger generation may wish to adhere to the traditions of their culture out of respect to relatives of an older generation.

Many cultures have deeply rooted belief systems that may compromise their acceptance of a Western medicine practice. For instance, in certain Asian cultures, herbs and acupuncture are first-line treatments for many ailments. Asians may fill a prescription so as not to insult the pharmacist or physician but never intend to actually take the medication. Or, they may fill a prescription, take it, and also take their trusted herbal remedy, which may interact with the medication. Being aware of the potential conflict between belief systems helps in identifying roadblocks that may contribute to the lack of a result from a medication or to uncommon toxicities.

Life-cycle rituals are also an area of vast cultural differences. Birth and death are two areas that directly affect health care delivery. For instance, in Hispanic cultures, large extended families expect to follow prospective mothers into the delivery room. This practice might be disconcerting to those with the traditional modesty values of American culture. Nonetheless, health care practitioners need to weigh the risk—that is, infection or hindrance of the provision of health care services—with the benefit of the patient's comfort and ease. While it is not necessarily the best idea to alter policy for every request, accommodating certain requests from patients may lead to better outcomes. Patients' attitudes have been shown to correlate with procedural and therapeutic outcomes.[2]

In American Indian culture, the ritual burial of the placenta is important. However, most hospitals routinely discard the placenta. The sensitive health care professional will make arrangements to provide the placenta to the family when asked.

A third example of a cultural issue regarding birth is the ritual circumcision on the eighth day of life of a Jewish boy. For most hospitals, circumcision is provided with parental consent before the family leaves the hospital. Wording a question ambiguously such as, "Do you want a circumcision for your son?" rather than, "Do you want a circumcision for your son in the hospital?" may result in the procedure being performed too early for Jewish practice.

Many cultures have deeply rooted belief systems that may compromise their acceptance of a Western medicine practice.

Language and Communication Styles

In English, *nova* refers to a star that suddenly becomes brighter. In Spanish, *no va* means "no go." In Vietnamese, the same two letters together can have multiple meanings depending on where the accent is placed in pronouncing the word. The slight mispronunciation of a patient's name or a word might mean something different—and possibly rude—in another language.

Gestures or body language can also have different meanings. In American culture, a handshake is considered a friendly business gesture, but in some other cultures, offering a hand to a stranger of the opposite sex is seen as inappropriate touching. In American culture, eye contact is considered polite, but in some Asian cultures, it would be considered forward and rude. Thus, to build and maintain rapport with customers, it is essential to become familiar with the communication styles of people who are patients in the business area where you work.

Cultural Differences in Pharmacy Situations

Let's examine some situations where cultural differences may affect interactions in the pharmacy. In American culture, we are used to addressing people by a title and surname, especially when speaking to elders. However, certain cultures find it disrespectful for someone unknown to the family or individual to address elders directly. (In fact, the Japanese have a different term for *mother* when it is used to refer to someone other than a person's own mother.) If you are working in an area with a lot of Japanese people and an elderly person comes in with a younger one, it may be appropriate to acknowledge the elder with a slight bow or nod and speak directly to the younger one.

As Americans, we are accustomed to being treated by professionals of either sex. In some cultures, treatment by someone of the opposite sex is considered taboo. It is not a question of equal rights but a question of sensitivity, comfort, and respect.

Americans feel strongly that adults are entitled to make their own decisions regarding health care issues and that patients should be given sufficient information regarding procedures to make informed decisions. Some Hispanic cultures rely heavily on the eldest son to make those decisions for parents. Other cultures may refer all treatment decisions to the parents regardless of the age of the patient. In others, an elder of the community is consulted for all essential decisions. This norm may delay a procedure or a decision while the appropriate person or persons are gathered.

Another way cultures differ is in the degree to which patients or close relatives are informed regarding a procedure. In some cultures, certain relatives, as well as even the patient, are only told that the patient is ill and are not informed of the diagnosis. Others may want the patient to know but not the children or the spouse. While health care providers have a duty to inform patients, it is also the prerogative of patients to make known their wishes regarding who has access to personal health information and who does not. If a patient asks you to follow a directive that is outside the norm and the request is documented, you can and should accommodate the request as long as no laws are broken.

Other cultural differences include beliefs in non-Western cures, commonly referred to as "complementary and alternative medicine." You may encounter a patient who believes in spiritual healing before, after, or concurrent with Western medicines. It is important to be respectful of these beliefs even when you cannot be a part of them. Sometimes, you need to accept that the patient is going to use complementary medications and make dose adjustments of Western medications rather than deny that the patient is doing so or insist that the patient stop. Of course, if the practice is dangerous, the patient must be advised about the consequences of continuing with a particular practice.

Patients need to feel comfortable with all health care practitioners, including technicians, so that they share all pertinent information. This requires that health care practitioners act nonjudgmentally and be open minded. It does not mean health care practitioners need to change their own beliefs.

You cannot assume that just because people appear to come from a particular culture, they subscribe to all the customs and beliefs of that culture.

Incorporating Knowledge into Practice

With these differences in mind, how do you handle the needs of a diverse population? First, you cannot assume that just because people appear to come from a particular culture, they subscribe to all the customs and beliefs of that culture. You need to be aware of the differences yet at the same time consider the degree to which individual members of a group have assimilated. Sometimes, asking directly is the best way to find out how someone wants to be treated. It can also be helpful to observe how a person relates to others in the group to learn whether traditional intergenerational signs of respect are followed.

Second, being respectful and knowledgeable does not mean that the health care team needs to be submissive to all demands from patients. Sometimes, it's appropriate to go along with a patient's culture. Sometimes, you must help the patient adapt American norms to his or her culture. Other times, you must politely but firmly hold your position.

In cases where the decision maker defined by the culture is not the patient, you can work with the family and the patient by having the patient formally designate a decision maker. The patient can either sign a formal document called a durable power of attorney or sign an acknowledgment that personal health care information will be shared with the designated person or persons the patient names. In cases where mind-altering agents are part of a spiritual healing ceremony, you can request that the ceremony be performed without these agents. Regardless of the extent to which an accommodation is possible, it is still appropriate to acknowledge the patient's right to hold to a belief or practice.

Patients with Physical Challenges

Many patients have physical challenges, such as blindness, immobility, a need for braces, or a hearing impairment. A physical handicap is not a reflection of a person's mental capacity. Patients facing physical difficulties deserve the same kindness and caring as patients without such challenges. Some people with physical handicaps appreciate offers of help and will take advantage of them. Others find that such offers, though intended in kindness, inhibit their sense of independence and self-reliance.

Not all people with handicaps and handicap stickers on their vehicles are confined to wheelchairs or use walkers to get around. Some physical handicaps may not be immediately noticeable. A person with a degenerative disease such as multiple sclerosis or someone with heart disease may not be able to stand for a long time or may have rested all day just to be able to walk to the pharmacy. Arthritic patients may have difficulty opening lids, but the affected joint, such as a wrist, might be covered. People in pain may do well for short periods but become disagreeable as their pain intensifies.

You must be sensitive to all people with physical challenges and be willing to accommodate them as much as possible. Sometimes, this means simply offering a chair. Sometimes, it means providing an accurate estimate of the wait time. It may even mean helping someone to the car or offering curbside service to someone who finds getting out of the car and coming into the pharmacy a hardship.

Working Animals

Guide dogs are assistants to people who are blind or physically challenged. Even in places where pets are unwelcome, guide dogs are allowed because they are working animals. Guide dogs provide eyes for the blind or mobility for the physically challenged. They give people independence.

Guide dogs are specially trained to behave certain ways in different circumstances. Unlike pets, they won't go up to strangers uninvited. Because guide dogs perform functions that their owners cannot, it is important to get permission from owners before petting or playing with their dogs. Of course, it would be inappropriate to do so when a blind person is being escorted across the street or when the dog is retrieving something for a wheelchair-bound person. A guide dog usually sits quietly under a table or under the seat of its owner's chair when it is not actively assisting.

Generally if the dog is with the owner in a public place, it is working. You need to respect that and not interfere with the working relationship unless you have permission. You don't want to distract an animal from the service it is performing. Fortunately, working animals often wear small coats that say they are guide dogs and not to pet them, so you will know not to request that they stay outside.

You may also encounter healing animals. These specially trained dogs, small horses, and other animals are used to bring comfort to hospitalized patients and patients in long-term care facilities. Some patients who have lost the ability to interact with other people, such as those with dementia, can still relate to animals. Children in hospitals respond positively to animal visitors as well. Some people with emotional issues may have their own comfort companions, as these animals are called. Understand that these animals are working, so you should ask the trainer or owner if it is acceptable to pet the animal before you do so. More often than not with comfort companions, petting is encouraged.

Patients facing physical difficulties deserve the same kindness and caring as patients without such challenges.

Visual Impairments and Blindness

When dealing with people who have visual disabilities, you may need to make accommodations. For partially sighted people, color coding with a marking pen may be sufficient to allow them to tell the difference between prescription medications. You might also write in large print the first letter of the name of each medication on each label. Unless the caps of the bottles are different sizes, placing identifiers only on the caps can lead to grave errors because they can inadvertently be placed on the wrong containers. Using different-size bottles and vials, even if all the medications fit into containers of the same size, is another method to help visually impaired patients distinguish medications.

You might also verbally describe the shape of each medication. As long as the shapes are significantly different, the patient will be able to tell them apart. For a partially sighted patient with diabetes, for example, you might describe glipizide as the smaller round tablet and metformin as the larger round tablet, since of the two white tablets, metformin is quite a bit larger. Or, one tablet might be oblong and the other round or flatter on one side. A blind person probably could not differentiate glipizide from baby aspirin, however, because the color difference between white and light orange is slight, and the sizes are similar. It's a good idea to ask patients what they find most helpful. Since most pharmacies are not able to type in Braille or get Braille translations of patient information sheets, it's especially important to give patients all necessary information clearly and slowly so that they can remember it.

Being observant and greeting the patient with a verbal explanation of what might otherwise be easily observed is often helpful. You might say, "Mr. Jones, how are you? We have several people waiting in front of you." Most blind people have assistants, guide dogs, or canes to make maneuvering easier. This does not mean that you can't offer to help or that you shouldn't explain that a door opens in (or out) when it's perhaps different from what would be expected. At the same time, try not to be overly solicitous.

Hearing Impairments and Deafness

People who are hearing impaired have special needs as well. For people who have acquired deafness, such as those who have become hard of hearing through age or because of illness or an accident, English is often a native language. If you cannot communicate verbally because you would need to be too loud or the person has such difficulty hearing that most of what you say would be lost, written communication is usually effective. Write the information in English no differently than you write or speak to anyone in everyday conversation. Since writing takes longer than speaking, be aware of lines that may build up and try to be efficient without making the person feel uncomfortable and rushed.

Some deaf people are keen lip readers and may ask you to communicate verbally. In this case, make sure you are facing the person and that you pronounce everything clearly. Remember that if you turn your head, the conversation automatically stops.

People who are born deaf have a unique form of communication. While American Sign Language (ASL) components can be learned by anyone, people who are born deaf may not have been educated in English as you know it. For them, sentence structure and the expression of an idea in ASL are completely different from what they are in English. Therefore, writing an English sentence instead of using sign language may be insufficient to communicate an idea. If you find that a simple written sentence seems to confuse a deaf person, try restructuring or rewording the idea. This may help convey the idea more easily. Pictures may also be effective.

You can also offer to provide a sign-language interpreter. This is optimal for complete understanding but may be impractical logistically. The Americans with Disabilities Act requires that a business obtain an interpreter if a deaf person requests one. A business is not required to retain an interpreter on site, so it may take some time to bring one in. The interpreter is paid either with public funds or by the business, depending on the jurisdiction and the location.

Besides a sign-language interpreter, another option for communicating with deaf and other hearing-impaired people is a telecommunications device for the deaf, or TDD. A TDD is a typewriter that converts spoken words into written words and is operated remotely via the telephone.

TDDs and sign-language interpreters are bound by law to translate verbatim. This means that sidebar conversations—those occurring with other people while you are waiting for the translator to finish translating what you just said—must be translated as well. So are words you wish you hadn't said, including expletives. The contents of sidebar conversations or inappropriate language can be distracting because the insertion of these comments may make it difficult to follow the conversation being translated. Unrelated comments or side comments can be taken the wrong way or be offensive, so be sure to stick with the main points and avoid excess conversation when you are working with a translator. In situations involving a translator or a TDD, it is a good idea to ask for frequent feedback to make sure the points you want to get across are being communicated correctly.

To facilitate transactions, deaf patients often bring family members along to translate what you say into sign language. While this may be helpful in some conversations, it may inhibit those involving sensitive or personal subjects. In addition, when difficult subjects are being discussed, interpreters who are family members may consciously or unconsciously insert their biases. Therefore, when possible, an impartial interpreter is a better option than a family member or friend. The same is also true for a patient who speaks a foreign language, although no law requires the provision of an unbiased translator when a person does not speak English.

Table 4-2 summarizes important guidelines for working with patients who have physical disabilities.

TABLE 4-2
Guidelines for Dealing with Patients with Physical Disabilities

▌ Ask people how they prefer to be accommodated.
▌ Offer to help. Don't assume that everyone in a wheelchair wants to be pushed.
▌ Use the words the patient uses to describe the disability. Ask if you don't know.
▌ Offer suggestions for what might help if the patient doesn't suggest something.

Political Correctness and Language Choices

Political correctness is not cultural competence. Some people do not favor the so-called acceptable language that is applied to them and their groups. The following story is an example.

Many years ago, two people were working closely together on a project. After some time, the sighted one asked the one who was using a machine that translated printed words into Braille what the correct terminology was for his condition. He answered, "I'm blind. I've been blind since birth. When you can't see, you're blind." Obviously, this person had no issue with the common English word and did not prefer the term *visually impaired* as a description of his blindness. Likewise, deaf people refer to their culture as deaf, not as hearing impaired.

The use of common English is intended to express an idea in a way that allows another to correctly receive a message. Blind means you can't see, and deaf means you can't hear. People with partial deficits may use terms such as partially blind, legally blind, or hearing impaired. For people without disabilities, the acknowledgment of a disability may make them uncomfortable. However, the reality is that many patients have handicaps that bear mentioning. When you are unsure about how to refer to a condition, ask the person what he or she prefers. Remember, though, that it is inappropriate to use slang terms that may be considered derogatory to describe a patient or a patient's condition. After all, you would not refer to the wife of a patient as the patient's "old lady." Dealing successfully with sensitivities such as cultural or physical differences depends on being aware and knowledgeable and displaying respect for patients and clients.

Dealing successfully with sensitivities such as cultural or physical differences depends on being aware and knowledgeable and displaying respect for patients and clients.

Religion

It has often been said that you can argue with a person's logic and you can disagree with a person's opinion, but when it comes to faith, all you can do is respect it. Faith and religion are expressions of spirituality. Thus, they may not seem to be based on reason or on fact. Instead, they are simply accepted. Religion holds tremendous power over people and can provide an unparalleled sense of peace to people of any faith. Spiritual beliefs are equally engaging.

Health care providers often need to make accommodations for religious practices. It is widely accepted that sick people are entitled and even encouraged to visit with a chaplain. In Western cultures, however, it is often less acceptable when a patient requests a shaman or some other healer. Health care practitioners who understand the healing capabilities of a blood transfusion may disapprove of members of Jehovah's Witnesses because they do not believe in sharing blood products. Some staff may find it odd that a follower of Islam requests a carpet on which to pray five times a day or that a Jewish person forbids the use of pork-based medication or sutures. Remember, your job is to heal and comfort, not to judge or ridicule.

Health care providers need to understand the importance of religious requests and try to accommodate them. A person's mind-set is as important to recovery as are the right diagnosis and medication. You need to respect these needs in the same way you respect the traditions of other cultures and the needs of people with disabilities.

You also need to afford patients the necessary time to perform rituals, unless they directly interfere with care. This may mean returning in 15 to 20 minutes to take vital signs so that an observant Jew can finish the Ma'ariv (evening) service. It may mean filling one prescription before another to allow someone to leave before sundown or in time for Ramadan study. It may mean arranging for kosher food trays for some patients or finding a nonbeef source of a medication for a strict Hindu.

Learning about Other Cultures

We have explored the ethnic, physical, religious, and cultural differences among people. How do you learn how to take care of a diverse population of patients?

One of the easiest ways to find out how to make people feel comfortable outside their familiar environments is to ask them. By asking, you may discover that some don't follow the rules of their ethnic groups. You may also learn that they follow customs you do not know about.

For instance, suppose you know that Jewish dietary laws prohibit eating shellfish and pork, so you order a vegetarian plate for a Jewish friend. Judaism has at least four "sects." Orthodox and some Conservative Jews keep the dietary laws, but few others do. You might learn that your Reform Jewish friend loves shrimp! Or, you may have read that Mormons don't drink alcohol or caffeinated beverages. Out of respect, you refrain from offering coffee to a patient only to find out that he enjoys two or three cups of coffee in the morning.

The best way to determine how to accommodate any particular patient's spiritual beliefs or rituals is to ask. By learning about different cultures, you become sensitive about when it is appropriate to ask. By asking, you show concern and respect for the person as an individual. After all, every culture has its rules. Every culture also has people who do not subscribe to them.

Another way to gain a deeper understanding of different cultures is through reading books and articles or attending classes. Just as there are dialects in some languages, sometimes there are local flavors to customs. These local customs may reflect different religious practices, or they may have evolved from necessity or convenience. A tradition resulting from a practical consideration, for instance, might be the staple in the main course for a feast. For seaside members of the culture, the entrée might be a marinated fish dish, while for those residing inland, it might feature lamb. Taking courses on all cultures is impractical, but it might be worthwhile to learn about the most common cultures of patients who frequent your pharmacy practice site.

A few books that discuss certain health-related customs of different cultures are available, but cultural reference books of any sort contain only snapshots of their subjects. As an overview, these books are a good beginning, but learning how a custom is practiced by the individual with whom you are working is best done by asking the person directly. Most people will be flattered that you have taken the initiative to become more familiar with their culture.

Traveling and going to museums are good ways to learn about different cultures. Through travel, you can see particular practices being performed directly by the very peoples who celebrate them. Visiting museums obviously is a less expensive and less time-consuming way to learn about cultures. Museums may have exhibitions that help explain rituals and customs. Frequently, museums that have cultural exhibitions also have guest lecturers to talk about the customs. Most of these lecturers also take questions or stay after they speak to chat awhile.

Resolving Cultural Conflicts

Cultural conflicts differ from other kinds of conflict in that the issues they call into question are core values. When you ask if someone would prefer a pen or pencil, emotion in the answer is unlikely. If you are serving coffee and ask, "Cream or sugar?" the person answers with a personal preference.

It is both courteous and wise to engage the patient in the resolution of an issue.

But when you suggest to a practicing Muslim who is fasting during Ramadan that he or she might want to get lunch while you fill the prescription, you offend the person's sensibilities. Knowing a bit about the culture enables you to make a better suggestion, such as, "Why don't you browse around, and your prescription will be ready in 15 minutes?"

When you comment that someone has a beautiful bracelet or a nice sweater, the person thinks you have good taste. When you say that someone looks well, it is taken as a sign that you are attentive and caring. When you notice bruises on a child's back and ask about them, you may just be expressing concern, but for people from certain Southeast Asian cultures, your concern may be taken as inappropriate or accusatory. The bruises could have been caused by coining, a traditional method of fighting disease. To avoid missteps, it is important that you become aware of practices different from your own. Apologize quickly if you inadvertently offend.

Where cultural practice clashes with treatment guidelines, it is both courteous and wise to engage the patient in the resolution of an issue. By inviting the patient's input, the resolution can address that patient needs. The health care professional can work with what is offered to ensure that the patient is cared for without compromising health care delivery or the laws and regulations governing the practice of pharmacy. Such an approach affords the greatest chance of the patient's compliance over the course of the treatment.

The dialogue can start with you simply asking, "What would work for you?" If the idea that is offered is not something that will work for the pharmacy, you can amend it, working toward a win-win solution. Another way to approach patient participation is to offer two or more alternatives that you can accept and allow the patient to pick the preferred one.

Summary

▌ Cultural competence starts by treating everyone with respect and as individuals.
▌ Asking patients how you can help in accommodating them shows concern.
▌ Considering patients' spiritual, cultural, and physical needs is as much a part of the treatment plan as the medical care is.

■ Patient-initiated ideas generally have the best chance of success.

■ Dealing with different cultures and sensitivities can be learned from classes, travel, museums, books, and interviews.

ACTIVITIES

1. Write a two-paragraph essay about your culture's approach to health care.

2. Hold a small-group discussion about health care differences in one another's families.

3. Hold a health care diversity awareness fair at your school.

4. Attend a religious service of an unfamiliar faith.

5. Interview people with backgrounds different from your own.

References

1. *Dictionary.com Unabridged (v. 1.1)*. Random House, Inc. http:// dictionary.reference.com/browse/culture (accessed November 17, 2008).

2. Cooper AF. Whose illness is it anyway? Why patient perceptions matter. *Int J Clin Pract*. 1998;52(8):551–6.

For More Information

Jacobson J. Counseling the deaf and hearing impaired. *Am J Health Syst Pharm*. 1999;56(7):610–1.

Lassiter SM. *Multicultural Clients: A Professional Handbook for Health Care Providers and Social Workers*. Westport, Conn: Greenwood Press; 1995.

Rundle A, Carvalho M, Robinson M. *Cultural Competence in Health Care: A Practical Guide*. San Francisco: Jossey-Bass; 2002.

Gardenswartz L, Rowe A. *Managing Diversity in Health Care: Proven Tools and Activities for Leaders and Trainers*. San Francisco: Jossey-Bass; 1998.

Searight HR, Gafford J. Cultural diversity and the end of life: issues and guidelines for the family physician. *Am Fam Physician*. 2005;71(3):515–22.

CHAPTER | 5

Professionalism and Ethics in the Workplace

Being professional and being ethical are important to maintaining the confidence that the public has in pharmacists and the people who work in pharmacies. Public relations is often thought of as the key to business success. Every employee working in a pharmacy is perceived by the public as an ambassador of that business. A good impression is equivalent to a single advertisement, but a poor image is almost impossible to shed. Therefore, all employees, no matter what their positions in the company's hierarchy, must understand that if any of the positions were not important, they would have been eliminated. In addition, all actions that employees take while at work create the overall perception the public has of the business.

Professionalism is determined by how we look and how we act. Like it or not, we make decisions about whether we want to associate with someone by how they appear. After the first impression and once people get to know one another, "company dress" is less important. Although friends and family may know you and appreciate your distinctive personality and many virtues, in the business world some level of conformity is expected. Clients and patients choose services from businesses that they perceive as maintaining certain standards. The first way to convey business competence is through your image, and image is determined by your appearance and your actions.

Put a different way, how appetizing would a restaurant be if the hostess had dirty fingernails, the waitress constantly scratched her arm, and the busboy looked like he had just finished changing the oil in his car? How much confidence would you have in a banker who wore a torn T-shirt and cutoffs and had a stale half-eaten bagel on his desk? Would you hire an attorney who had a small basketball hoop in his office and "shot a few" while he listened to your case?

The answer is obvious. Now think about the fact that you are working in an environment where people trust you with

Professionalism is determined by how we look and how we act.

one of their most valuable assets—their health. They want to know that they can trust what you say, what you do, and what you prepare for them. Developing this confidence in an impersonal world is done by living up to or exceeding the image patients have for the person doing the job. In pharmacy, confidence is built by looking like a professional and acting like one.

The first rule of professionalism is fundamental cleanliness and presentation. It is important to be well groomed and relatively conservative in dress. Coming to work looking disheveled sends a message to your boss that you don't value your position. It also sends a message to patients and other customers that you don't care and, by association, neither does the business.

Cleanliness and modest makeup are preferred business grooming. Makeup should be worn to enhance features, not to make a statement. Remember, you are working close to people, so heavy makeup will appear overdone. Conservative tones are more businesslike than bright colors. The same is true of hair tones. Hair should be styled in a manner that allows your eyes to be seen and that gives you freedom of movement without it becoming untidy or "coming down" if you bend down. If you tend to fidget with your hair, find a way to keep it back so you are not tempted to play with it while talking with a patient or pharmacist.

A daily shower or bath, as well as deodorant, is standard. Being malodorous disturbs your fellow technicians and pharmacists, offends patients, and makes for an uncomfortable conversation with your supervisor. In most cases, light or no perfume should be used, since many people are allergic to scents. Moreover, strong scents are not perceived the same way by all noses. What appeals to one person may smell like a moldy attic to another. In a small area, a strong, sweet scent can become unpleasant over time. A rule of thumb regarding perfume is that if you can smell your own, it's too much.

Standard pharmacy dress for men is slacks—not jeans—and a shirt. Many businesses prefer button shirts, but in some places, golf shirts are allowed. Some venues require ties as well. These may be colorful and creative, but they should not serve as billboards for political agendas of any sort. T-shirts of any kind should not be worn in a pharmacy unless it is a nonpublic compounding type of pharmacy. Unless issued by the organization in which you are working, logo wear is inappropriate. Even when you work in a compounding or sterile-product area where you change into scrubs, if you need to walk through public areas of the building or hospital before and after work, it is preferable that you blend in with the clientele or the business image.

Similarly, women should be presentable when walking in public places whether or not a uniform is required at work. For nonuniform positions, slacks or skirts and business tops are appropriate. Dresses may also be worn, keeping in mind that you will frequently be bending and moving about. Therefore, a skirt of modest length that affords flexibility without being revealing is preferred. Shirts or blouses that show the midriff are not acceptable in a business environment. Neither are low-cut, sheer, or otherwise provocative tops. Again, like men, you are not a human billboard, so logo wear of any business other than the one you work in is inappropriate. Suits may be worn by either sex, although in most patient-care pharmacy areas, suits are considered a little too formal.

Hose or socks should be worn with closed-toe and closed-back shoes. A heel height that allows you to stand comfortably for long periods is also helpful. Jewelry should be tasteful and not get in the way of job function. Shoes for either male or female employees should be clean, polished, and in good repair.

Hands and nails are an important part of grooming too. Because a handshake is still the conventional business greeting, hands are often on display. They should be smooth and clean. Nails should be relatively short, since long nails can harbor germs. Although you will wear gloves in most sterile manufacturing and compounding areas, jobs involving a lot of sterile compounding may require that you not have any type of artificial nails. This is a direct outcome from the Centers for Disease Control and Prevention's recommendations published in 2002.[1] No subsequent guidelines have been published. In addition, there are no data to refute or support the necessity of not having artificial nails in light of the use of gloves for patient care and for sterile manufacturing. Washing your hands between patients and before regloving is a good hygiene and safety practice. Such a great amount of hand washing can leave hands rough, so applying a good lotion is often essential.

Like the overall first impression, a handshake is often a bond builder or deal breaker. If you wear polish, it should not be chipped. A handshake should be firm, not too long, and not too tight. Offering your hand first is a gesture of friendliness and should be accompanied by making eye contact.

You may also use your hand to reassure a patient or family member. You can offer your hands to support a patient or to steady someone getting up. Your hands also are on display when you give someone a medication, take in a prescription, lend a pen, or direct someone to another area.

Whether you wear a smock or lab coat depends on the supervisor of your pharmacy. In some practice sites, a lab coat signifies a professional, such as a pharmacist or doctor. In some institutions, short coats signify interns or trainees, and fingertip-length coats are reserved for degreed and licensed personnel. If your place of practice puts ranks on the coats, then it is inappropriate for you to wear one. But if technicians wear short coats and pharmacists wear long ones, then the norm would be appropriate.

Table 5-1 summarizes the do's and don'ts of attire in the workplace.

TABLE 5-1

Do's and Don'ts of Professional Attire

- Do wear wrinkle-free or neatly pressed slacks, skirts, and blouses or shirts.
- Do wear closed-toe shoes.
- Do wear hose without holes and in a color that complements the outfit.
- Do have a neatly styled haircut that is easy to maintain during the workday.
- Do shower or bathe before the start of each workday.
- Do wear a conservative amount of makeup in relatively natural-looking colors.
- Don't wear clothing that allows undergarments to show.
- Don't assume that a lab coat will cover a wrinkled or unclean, casual appearance.
- Don't wear dramatic makeup.
- Do wear clothing that allows you to bend, stand on your toes, and move comfortably.
- Don't wear flip-flops.
- Don't wear fabrics that are too clingy or too sheer.
- Don't wear logo attire unless it is issued by the operation where you work.

Who Are Your Customers?

When we talk about professionalism, does that mean being professional only with other professionals? Whose respect are we trying to cultivate anyway?

Let's consider who the customers are in any line of pharmacy work. Customers are people interacting with you and the pharmacists during the course of the business day. In general, a business considers those who are in a position to form an opinion that can affect the business to be customers.

Obviously, patients and their families are customers. Whoever comes to pick up a prescription, inquire about over-the-counter medications, accompany a patient, or shop in the store where the pharmacy is located is a customer. Everybody who makes contact is a potential pharmacy patron even if the immediate visit has nothing to do with a personal need for pharmacy services. Who knows who may be sick or need preventative medications in the future? In addition, doctors, nurses, and other health care providers are customers in the sense that the pharmacy provides a service to them. The service could be answering a question, sharing a patient, providing a medication, or giving advice.

Depending on who your employer is, pharmacists may be your customers. If you are working in a warehouse of some sort or in an outsourced pharmacy that provides services such as sterile-product admixtures or nuclear pharmaceuticals to pharmacies, pharmacists are certainly your customers. Technicians working in a pharmacy benefit management business also have pharmacists as customers. Technicians working in the business aspect of any pharmacy may have business executives, managers, accountants, clerks, insurance adjusters, and pharmacy benefit managers as customers. People working in a hospital setting or for a chain drugstore may have corporate office employees as customers. Table 5-2 lists some of the many categories of people who are pharmacy customers.

TABLE 5-2

Who Are Pharmacy Customers?

- Patients
- Nurses
- Doctors
- Patients' families and friends
- Insurance company personnel
- Hospital administrators
- Pharmacy CEOs
- Businesses

Handle yourself with each patient or customer as though you were interacting with the most important person you can imagine.

Whether someone is a patient or not, your interaction should always be at a professional level. At work, decorum is important, and how you handle yourself with everyone—patient, client, customer, or anyone else—is likely to be witnessed and to make an impression on others. For this reason, it is essential that you handle yourself with each patient or customer as though you were interacting with the most important person you can imagine.

In addition to dress, demeanor is another measure of your professionalism. Have you ever entered a business only to be ignored by someone catching up on last night's gossip via the company phone? Do you remember feeling invisible to a service provider who seemed more interested in stocking shelves than in giving assistance? Have you ever overheard two employees complaining about a customer or describing someone in negative terms? These are all examples of unprofessional behavior.

Professional conduct shows observers that you respect your surroundings and you respect your patients and customers. You can easily reinforce your professional image in a couple of ways.

Posture is important. If possible, stand and sit straight. Your mother was right when she suggested that sitting slumped in a chair makes you look like a tired piece of cloth, not an energetic, helpful person. Good posture conveys a sense of self-respect. It also conveys a sense of openness and a willingness to assist people.

Making yourself aware of your surroundings and particularly the people in it is another way to support a professional image. Scanning your pharmacy environment at frequent intervals provides you with the opportunity to greet newcomers soon after their arrival with at least a friendly, "Hello, I'll be right with you." Everyone is busy in today's understaffed, overworked world. (It's not entirely true, but we've all had "those days" often enough.) Even so, unless you just engaged in activity with another patient, excuse yourself from the first conversation to acknowledge a newcomer. If you can predict about how long the wait might be, it is appropriate to mention that as well.

Managing your interaction with customers is also important. When a long-winded and frequent patient or customer comes to your pharmacy on a busy day, place a limit on your conversation ahead of time. You can do this through a comment such as, "Hi, Mrs. Bloom. It's good to see you. It's awfully busy today. What can I do for you?" This communicates in advance that you won't have a lot of time for conversation. If others start to line up or you simply must get back to the work at hand, ask permission to move on after you've finished the business part of the visit. You might say, "I'd love to hear more about that, but right now, I should help the gentleman behind you," or, "It's good to see you. You won't mind if I get back to filling these orders [or finishing this report] before I fall further behind, will you?"

Table 5-3 summarizes some key elements for evaluating professionalism.

TABLE 5-3
How to Measure a Professional

▌ Dress
▌ Cleanliness
▌ Attitude
▌ Voice tone
▌ Work ethic
▌ Attention to detail
▌ Persistence to the task at hand

Greeting Patients

The welcome is an important step in engaging a patient or pharmacy customer. People should be acknowledged as soon as they enter the space in which you can reasonably interact with them. Even if you are on the phone with a patient or customer, nodding your head to newcomers goes a long way toward calming them and assuring them that you will get to them as soon as possible.

You can also convey a welcome with a smile, the words *welcome* or *hello,* or a question such as, "How may I assist you?" The question "Whaddaya want?" is not a professional greeting. Neither is a grunt disguised as a greeting. Continuing to bow your head and work on a task convinces no one that you did not see the newest customer, doctor, nurse, or other co-worker.

Once you greet people, it is important to address their concerns as soon as possible. If you see a newcomer to the operation near the area where you are, you might volunteer to help out if possible. This can easily be done in a small satellite pharmacy, since nurses and doctors come sporadically. In a larger retail pharmacy, patients arrive in a more constant flow, so allowing a small line to develop is not unreasonable. Even in such a setting, however, if one patient or client is taking up an inordinate amount of time, it would not be unreasonable for another staff member to take care of the waiters and then resume normal chores. If a second staff member is not available to help, it is also not unreasonable to ask the patient if you could be excused to help the "quickies"—but only if the transaction is exceptionally lengthy.

What is most important to remember as a professional is that the customers, patients, and clients *are* the reason you are there. They are *not* the interruptions that interfere with getting your work done. Were it not for the human beings in need of every order you fill or every prescription you take in, you would have no work to get done. As an employee, you must develop the skill to work efficiently and in such a way as to finish routine tasks in between taking care of "live" or "walk-up" customers. It is up to the manager to employ enough staff to take care of routine business efficiently and maintain and service the customers and patients. It is also up to the manager to work out a schedule that puts enough people in the pharmacy at times when it is busiest.

Empathy, Sympathy, and Other Expressions

Professionalism is also how you say things and your non-verbal communication. Conducting yourself as a professional means being empathetic and sympathetic, as well as being a coach who may deliver information that the patient does not want to hear. Sympathy and empathy entail listening attentively to stories that may not interest you. It also means recognizing when a person may need extra reassurance. Sometimes it means giving someone space. In the pharmacy world, people often share things that are personal. It is important to listen when appropriate and to learn how to graciously end a conversation that is either inappropriate or that is taking up too much of your time.

One of the signs of being a professional is recognizing that you do not know everything.

Professionalism and Patient Confidentiality

People tell health care providers all kinds of stories. Sometimes they share something because they are lonely. Other times, they have no one else to turn to. Sometimes they are scared or confused. It's your job to help reassure, educate, and console. Some of these emotions can be eased by an understanding technician, but other times the patient needs to be referred to a pharmacist because the pharmacist is best able to handle the patient's concern or because the patient is requesting advice. Regardless of how entertaining the story might be, tales from the trenches should not be shared at parties, with close friends, or at dinner. The adage "You never know who knows who" particularly applies in these situations.

For information on the confidentiality of patients' private health information and the Health Insurance Portability and Accountability Act (HIPAA), see Chapter 6.

Answering Difficult Questions

One of the signs of being a professional is recognizing that you do not know everything. It is perfectly acceptable to say that you need to consult someone else or check the facts. Make sure, however, that you get back to the person even if it is to say you need more time. You can also refer someone to a better resource, such as a pharmacist.

It is unprofessional to lie or make up an answer to appear knowledgeable. It is also unacceptable to tell patients or customers that you don't know and not follow up with a resource to find out. Besides referring patients to a pharmacist, you can direct them to employees in other departments. For instance, if a person asks about visiting hours and you don't know, you might send or take the person to the information desk. If someone is having an issue with a third-party payer, you might offer to dial the insurance claims department. If a person is looking for a location in the building that is unfamiliar to you, you might provide a map or offer to make a phone call.

Professional conduct involves problem solving. Although technicians perform tasks that do not involve professional judgment, acting like a professional is an asset to the organization and to yourself. When you deal with patients, ask yourself, "How would I like to be treated if I were in their workplace and needed assistance with a problem?" or, "If I needed this answer myself, how would I go about getting it?" This type of problem solving may sound a bit creative. The more information you accumulate as a result of experience, however, the better able you are to help people directly, and even if you can't, you are still better equipped to use your knowledge and skills to direct people to the correct source of the information.

Professional Image and the Office Party

Everyone wants to have fun. Many organizations have holiday parties or seasonal get-togethers that allow people to mingle and get to know one another outside the formality of the work environment. Nothing ruins more careers than poor behavior at an office get-together.

Remember that although it is a party, it is a work party. If the event takes place at your place of business and includes patients or customers, it is especially important that you maintain a work image, albeit a relaxed one. Even if the owner is telling off-color jokes or a key customer is drinking too much, the wise employee exercises restraint.

The saying "Loose lips sink ships" is particularly true in the work environment. Nothing loosens lips faster than alcohol. In social situations involving work, limit alcohol consumption to one less drink an hour than you know you can easily tolerate. If drinking excessively is a problem you have encountered before, then it is prudent to avoid alcohol altogether.

Like drinking excessively, telling crude and off-color stories is unacceptable. And gossip is not party conversation. Develop some topics you can offer as conversation starters. These might include vacations you have enjoyed or those someone else is going on, movies or other entertainment events, accomplishments of your colleagues you'd like to know more about, or current events. Avoid topics that can become emotional, and change subjects if someone is getting upset. While discussion of an issue is healthy, a fight is not what a party is all about.

Professionalism and Manners for the Workplace

Today, the term *rude* often refers to an attitude, not to an action. Traditional manners are often thought of as stuffy, and yet most of them have been developed to provide comfort to all individuals involved. Manners dictate expectations and allow people interacting with one another to anticipate what comes next. Despite the evolution of manners, there are some rules that need to be followed in the business setting.

Cell Phones and Pagers

Today, most people have cell phones, and inconsiderate behavior is often an unfortunate consequence. At work, a personal cell phone should be turned off or in the silent position. In most cases, keeping it in your locker or car is best. Unless you have some pressing need, calls should be received and returned after work. After all, you have been hired because the organization needs you to devote your attention and skills to it.

A pressing need is something that immediately affects health or quality of life—for example, a call about the outcome of a relative's surgery or a call from a physician about your health. In rare cases, it may involve a household emergency. Pressing issues do not include notification from your best friend about a sale at a favorite store or an announcement that concert tickets are available. It is most inappropriate to shout during a call taken at a business, whether it is a happy scream or one directed at misbehaving children.

For calls that you expect, it is best to let your supervisor know ahead of time. When a call comes, excuse yourself from the work area for a short period of time to answer it. If you are attending a meeting during which you expect a call, it is appropriate to let the other attendees know that you may be called away during the meeting.

For business-issued pagers, the protocol is different. Pagers are used by those in fields such as medicine who need to be contacted immediately about critical issues. Pages should be returned as soon as possible. Alpha pagers make returning calls easier because they can give you preliminary information about the matter and allow you to retrieve necessary files or other materials before returning the call. When you page others, using the alpha page option also allows them to be prepared. With alpha pagers, you can communicate whether or not immediate attention is necessary. For instance, you could page a doctor with a request such as, "Please confirm dose of propranolol on patient Morgan."

Taking Responsibility Is Part of Professionalism

Everyone makes mistakes. Professionals take responsibility for their actions. It is also a professional responsibility to try to make things work better and to work things out when they don't go as planned.

Mistakes occur for many reasons, but primarily they are "accidental"—that is, the people making them did so unintentionally. Although they are accidents, some errors are preventable. Sometimes an error is made because there is a flaw in the system. Errors of this nature can be prevented by adjusting the system in some way. For example, a double-check system might be put in place, adding another person or another step to a process. Sometimes errors occur because of insufficient training. For example, a lack of knowledge might lead a technician to mistake a new drug for a familiar one that looks and sounds similar. Some errors result from poor management. They are committed by staff but are really caused by understaffing or unreal expectations by management in terms of what can be done in a specified time frame. Finally, though, some mistakes occur no matter what anyone does.

When an error occurs, it is everyone's responsibility to learn from the mistake so that it does not get repeated. In some operations, near misses are reported so that teams can figure out ways to prevent even these from occurring. In the pharmacy world, a near miss is an error that is caught before it gets to the patient.

Besides figuring out how to prevent an error from recurring, errors that get to patients need to be reported to them. This allows patients to stop taking a medication that could cause damage. It can also inform them about what effects to watch for from an incorrect drug.

In the outpatient setting, patients may call to ask about the physical appearance of a medication. Nowadays, a description of the medication is required on the container in many states, although the print is small and difficult for some to read. When brands of generic drugs are switched, the computer is updated so that the description printed on the container is accurate. Nonetheless, when a patient calls about the accuracy of a prescription, it is always prudent to double-check in case an error has occurred. Even if the description on the container matches what is in it, an error may have been made in what was ordered or what was used to fill the prescription. It is better to be interrupted a hundred times and be right than it is to assume you are right and be wrong, especially if there are major ramifications. Always thank a person who calls to confirm a product, even when you are correct.

In the inpatient setting, patients are less likely to question medications. Still, patients are entitled to the five rights of medication: the right drug to the right patient at the right time in the right dosage form and dose.

If you make an error, apologize for it. Don't make excuses, and don't blame someone else for an error you made. Try to fix it as soon as possible. If you can think of ways to prevent the error in the future, share them with your boss. Finding better ways to do things is not the same as making excuses for an error because the fixes were not in place.

Some mistakes in the pharmacy setting do not involve medications. Sometimes errors in judgment or errors of omission occur. An error in judgment, for example, is holding rigorously to a policy where there is room for flexibility.

Patients are entitled to the five rights of medication: the right drug to the right patient at the right time in the right dosage form and dose.

Or a staff member might oversleep or get confused about a shift, inadvertently causing staffing problems. If the problem is an error in judgment or a recurring issue, the supervisor should discuss it with the staff member (see Chapter 11 on staff management). Errors of omission include forgetting to schedule someone, not placing an order when asked to, or forgetting to reconcile something. Correct the situation as soon as you are notified. If this means going in to work as soon as you are called, give a realistic time for when you can be there and make it happen.

Timeliness

Like taking responsibility for fixing errors, maintaining a commitment to timeliness reflects positively on your professionalism. Being at work on time is one aspect of this. If you get caught in traffic, admit it and try to determine alternate routes to work. If you are regularly late, promise to leave earlier in the future and do it. Empty promises and repeated excuses cause others to lose respect for you.

Similarly, timeliness is an issue with work assignments. Often when assigning reports or project work, a supervisor asks for a time frame in which to expect the finished product. In other cases, a deadline is given. When asked to estimate a time frame, consider what needs to be accomplished and give a realistic date for completion. Once you have estimated the time, do everything you can to meet the deadline or finish early. Regardless of how significant missing a deadline is, the inability to meet the deadline, self-imposed or otherwise, should be brought to the supervisor's attention as soon as it is known. This allows the supervisor to change the priorities, assign more staff to the project, or extend the deadline. Not mentioning it with the hope that no one will notice is unprofessional and often disappoints not only the boss who is expecting the work. Your project may be part of a larger project that depends on your work to move forward. In some cases, missed deadlines have financial consequences that you may not be aware of. Keeping the boss informed of progress avoids surprises and shows that you are responsible.

76 | Communication & Management Skills for the Pharmacy Technician

Meeting Manners

Another misstep that many people make in business is regularly showing up late to meetings. This is acceptable only if you work in direct patient care—and only once in a while. Keeping others waiting so you can catch up on something else is unacceptable. Asking people to repeat what occurred in your absence shows others that you value your time more than theirs.

If you are running a meeting, the most professional approach is to print an agenda ahead of time. An agenda informs participants about what is to be discussed and allows them to prepare. Including on the agenda an estimate of the amount of time that will be devoted to each topic is helpful. For example, updating everyone on work in progress should require less time than discussing a proposition that needs approval to go forward. Don't waste time reading something to participants that they can read themselves, but don't assume that everyone is up to speed on an important issue that has not been discussed.

Meetings should occur only when everyone's input is necessary or an announcement needs to be made in a way that ensures everyone hears it at the same time and understands it. Meetings can be run with one-way communication—that is, when the chairperson does most of the talking. It is then akin to a briefing session. Other meetings invite input and have multiple participants sharing ideas.

Regularly occurring meetings held with no purpose promote disrespect. If staff members are made to come to such meetings, they may tune out and miss an important issue. They may also start to plan conflicting appointments to avoid the meetings. Canceling too many routine meetings, however, invites mistrust as well. Why schedule a meeting if you have no intention of holding it? A good manager holds formal or informal staff meetings regularly so that both the manager and the staff are kept abreast of what is occurring in the organization. A manager has made a critical mistake if the staff must hear about important information from sources outside the department.

For additional information on meetings, see Chapter 12.

ACTIVITIES

1. Try on several types of clothing you own in front of a mirror. Which image would you be most comfortable approaching with a personal problem?

2. Visit a bank, a supermarket, a high-end department store, a standard department store, a discount clothing store, and four other types of businesses. What do you observe about the differences in dress? Which operations make you think "professional"?

3. When you observed the different businesses, what actions of particular employees made you want to do business with the store? Which actions turned you off?

4. Observe someone in a customer-service capacity for an hour. How does this person address customers? How does this person carry himself or herself? Would you want to respond the same way? How would you work differently with customers?

5. Think back to a school party you attended. Describe behavior you thought was positive.

6. Remember someone at a party who left a negative impression on you. What was it about his or her behavior that caused you to view this person less favorably?

Ethics

While professionalism has specific attributes, ethics are much more personal. Professional behavior is in part judged by others, and their perceptions—right or wrong—determine the acceptability of you as a technician or health care worker. A lack of acceptance can result in a business losing patients. The personal principles of ethics people adopt reflect who they are—their upbringing, religious affiliation, and core values—but cannot be easily identified from the outside. In addition to personal ethics, widely accepted professional ethics often guide workplace behavior. In the pharmacy world, for example, many organizations have developed codes of ethics for pharmacists and technicians. Like acting in an unprofessional manner, exhibiting questionable personal and professional ethics can lead to a loss of business.

Ethical behavior is shaped by basic values such as not stealing, treating others in an honest and respectful fashion, recognizing and respecting property that is not yours, and not being envious of the accomplishments and property of others. In some situations, the right path is obvious, but there are many situations where it is less certain. In ethics, sometimes there are no right or wrong answers, just better options than others. Slight variations in situations may completely change how they are resolved. Let's look at how some of these values translate into ethical business practices.

In ethics, sometimes there are no right or wrong answers, just better options than others.

Situation 1

You and a colleague started working at the pharmacy on the same day. Several years have passed, and the two of you do similar work with a similar level of accuracy. Because you are friends, you have shared your evaluations and raises with each other, and you both have progressed at about the same rate.

A position that would be a small promotion is going to open at a new location. Only one of you can get it.

▮ The position would be a closer drive for you than for your friend, so you arrange for an opportunity to tell the boss. Is this ethical? Why or why not?

▮ The pharmacist working at the new location went out with your colleague many years ago. The relationship ended badly. Both went on to new relationships, however, and are married to other people. You tell the decision maker that this previous relationship may be a problem if the two are going to work together. Is this ethical? Why or why not?

▮ Your colleague once called in sick to go skiing. You know that the decision maker disapproves of lying. Since you want the job badly, you tell the decision maker, hoping this information will sway the job in your favor. Is this ethical? Why or why not?

▮ You find out that the job will be awarded in two weeks. You make an appointment with the decision maker and explain why you think you should get the job. Is this ethical? Why or why not? What if your colleague is away on vacation and can't make an appointment as well?

Situation 2

The pharmacist is going on a vacation and tells you that she can't sleep on planes. You notice that she writes a prescription for herself for five sleeping pills and uses the name of a doctor you know is her friend as the prescriber. The pharmacist asks you to type the prescription. She notes it as a verbal prescription, but you know there were no phone calls to the pharmacy. After the prescription is filled, the pharmacist pays for the medication.

- Is the pharmacist's conduct ethical? Why or why not? What action, if any, should you take?
- Would the situation be different if the sleeping pills are a controlled substance?
- What if the doctor wants to prescribe medication for himself, but because it is a controlled substance, he calls and asks the pharmacist to use her name as the patient. Is this ethical? Why or why not?
- Suppose the prescription is for a medication for someone with no insurance. The pharmacist uses her name because she has insurance. The patient pays the co-pay, and the rest is billed to the third party. Is this ethical? Why or why not?

Situation 3

You work in a pharmacy. Other employees expect the pharmacist to give them free medication when they forget to take their own at home or when they develop a symptom at work.

- The pharmacy is owned by a sole proprietor. Business is falling, but the pharmacist still wants to be a nice guy. Is this ethical? Why or why not?
- The pharmacy is in a large hospital. Volume is high, and the census is always near capacity. A few tablets will not be missed. Is this ethical? Why or why not?
- The person asking is a doctor who asks for medications at least once a week. She tells you that she could get samples anyway. Is this doctor being ethical? Why or why not? Is giving her a few doses ethical?

▌ An employee who never asks for free medication is suffering from an awful headache. If the pharmacist doesn't give him something for the symptoms, he will have to go home, leaving the operation short-staffed and increasing the workload of the rest of the staff. Is this ethical? Why or why not?

Situation 4

You work in a pharmacy that you like. Everyone is fun to work with. You know, however, that the prices are better down the street. You wonder if you should tell the patients.

▌ Some of your customers have limited resources. You send them to the other pharmacy when nobody can hear you. Is this ethical? Why or why not?

▌ An affluent patient complains about the prices. You send her to the other pharmacy. Is this ethical? Why or why not?

▌ A patient complains about the prices. You suggest he shop around. Is this ethical? Why or why not?

▌ You figure if people were concerned enough about the prices, they would shop around. You keep the information to yourself and assume it's the service or location that keeps the patients coming back. Is this ethical? Why or why not?

▌ People start transferring their prescriptions to the other pharmacy. The boss is concerned. You mention that the prices are better down the street and suggest that your pharmacy try to match them. Is this ethical? Why or why not?

Situation 5

Someone who doesn't use your pharmacy or hospital calls repeatedly to ask the pharmacist questions. Most of the time, the questions are complex and take at least 5 minutes to answer.

▌ Is the patient's conduct ethical? Why or why not?

▌ Does it matter if your pharmacy doesn't take the patient's health insurance?

▌ What if the person used to be a patient of your pharmacy?

▌ What, if anything, should the pharmacist say?

Ethics consider not only the person acting but also the good of the whole.

Situation 6

You have heard about an efficient pharmacy operation not too far away from your pharmacy. The pharmacist-in-charge at your pharmacy wants to find out how the other pharmacy is run.

▌ You get a part-time job at the other pharmacy with the intention of leaving in a few months after you learn about the operation. After all, you think, who couldn't use a little extra cash? Is this ethical? Why or why not?

▌ You call the other pharmacy pretending to be a patient. Is this ethical? Why or why not?

▌ You visit the other pharmacy and ask to speak with the person in charge. Then you explain what you want to know and ask if you can talk with him. Is this ethical? Why or why not?

Situation 7

Your friend gets tickets to a hot concert. You are scheduled to work the next day. The concert is several hours away, and the likelihood of your returning in time to get adequate rest is slim.

▌ The last time you asked a colleague to trade shifts with you, she couldn't do it. You decide to call in sick. After all, you think, you've earned it. Is this ethical? Why or why not?

▌ You explain the situation to the boss and promise to come in as soon as you wake up. Is this ethical? Why or why not?

▌ You ask to have the next day off. The boss explains that he can't give it to you, so you call in sick. Is this ethical? Why or why not?

Ethics determine the respectability of a business, but ethical behavior is governed by personal values of right and wrong. One gold standard is, Can you look yourself in the mirror tomorrow if you do what you are doing today? The Golden Rule—Do unto others as you would have them do unto you—is another standard of ethical behavior. These principles are similar, but are they practical? In a business setting, questions to think about include the following: Is the time you are asking someone to spend with you taking away from his or her productivity? Will tangible losses be sustained if the request is granted? Is the action going to increase the pharmacy's business or reputation in the long run even though it is going to cost now?

Ethics differs from law. Although law is based on ethical standards, illegal actions lead to consequences. Law has definite rights and wrongs—it is black and white. With ethics, rights and wrongs are gray. Even in the situations above, there may be exceptions to the standard "right" answers. In other words, in ethics there are no hard and fast rules. In similar situations, different circumstances may lead you to completely different answers.

What would happen if a person decided how to act solely by answering the question, "Why not do it, since I can and if I did, it wouldn't bother me?" Is it still the right thing to do if that individual is OK with the act? Sometimes it is, and sometimes it is not. What about a situation where the act would have undesirable consequences if someone found out, but the likelihood of it being discovered is slim? Ethics consider not only the person acting but also the good of the whole. Ethical behavior is governed by the belief that if something were found out, it would pass the decency test. Another way to refer to this is called the "sunshine rule"—if the action took place in broad daylight with everyone concerned around, would it appear to be ethical? If not, don't do it.

From the sunshine rule developed the disclosure rule. Many professionals felt that some speakers were subtly and not so subtly slanting their presentations toward particular drugs because they were funded by pharmaceutical companies. To address this ethical issue, the pharmaceutical industry, continuing-education providers, the American Medical Association, and pharmacy associations developed guidelines requiring disclosure of speakers' funding sources or sponsorships. The intent was to inform people about the possible biases of speakers and keep presentations open and informative.

Many pharmacy societies have developed their own codes of ethics for pharmacists and technicians. Figure 5-1 is the code of ethics from the American Pharmacists Association. This document was adapted by the American Association of Pharmacy Technicians, so its code is similar. Note that the code focuses on honesty, respect, and optimal therapy for all.

FIGURE 5-1

Code of Ethics for Pharmacists

Preamble

Pharmacists are health professionals who assist individuals in making the best use of medications. This Code, prepared and supported by pharmacists, is intended to state publicly the principles that form the fundamental basis of the roles and responsibilities of pharmacists. These principles, based on moral obligations and virtues, are established to guide pharmacists in relationships with patients, health professionals, and society.

I. A pharmacist respects the covenantal relationship between the patient and pharmacist.

Considering the patient-pharmacist relationship as a covenant means that a pharmacist has moral obligations in response to the gift of trust received from society. In return for this gift, a pharmacist promises to help individuals achieve optimum benefit from their medications, to be committed to their welfare, and to maintain their trust.

II. A pharmacist promotes the good of every patient in a caring, compassionate, and confidential manner.

A pharmacist places concern for the well-being of the patient at the center of professional practice. In doing so, a pharmacist considers needs stated by the patient as well as those defined by health science. A pharmacist is dedicated to protecting the dignity of the patient. With a caring attitude and a compassionate spirit, a pharmacist focuses on serving the patient in a private and confidential manner.

III. A pharmacist respects the autonomy and dignity of each patient.

A pharmacist promotes the right of self-determination and recognizes individual self-worth by encouraging patients to participate in decisions about their health. A pharmacist communicates with patients in terms that are understandable. In all cases, a pharmacist respects personal and cultural differences among patients.

IV. A pharmacist acts with honesty and integrity in professional relationships.

A pharmacist has a duty to tell the truth and to act with conviction of conscience. A pharmacist avoids discriminatory practices, behavior, or work conditions that impair professional judgment, and actions that compromise dedication to the best interests of patients.

FIGURE 5-1, continued

V. A pharmacist maintains professional competence.
A pharmacist has a duty to maintain knowledge and abilities as new medications, devices, and technologies become available and as health information advances.

VI. A pharmacist respects the values and abilities of colleagues and other health professionals.
When appropriate, a pharmacist asks for the consultation of colleagues or other health professionals or refers the patient. A pharmacist acknowledges that colleagues and other health professionals may differ in the beliefs and values they apply to the care of the patient.

VII. A pharmacist serves individual, community, and societal needs.
The primary obligation of a pharmacist is to individual patients. However, the obligations of a pharmacist may at times extend beyond the individual to the community and society. In these situations, the pharmacist recognizes the responsibilities that accompany these obligations and acts accordingly.

VIII. A pharmacist seeks justice in the distribution of health resources.
When health resources are allocated, a pharmacist is fair and equitable, balancing the needs of patients and society.

Adopted by the American Pharmacists Association membership, October 27, 1994.

Summary

▌ Professionalism is a code of conduct that gives an outward appearance to observers and customers. Professional behavior gives an air of importance and a sense of trust to an operation.

▌ Honesty and accountability are two important attributes of professional demeanor.

▌ Ethics is a set of personal principles that guide a person in making decisions. These principles are based on religious teaching, community morals, and upbringing.

Reference

1. Centers for Disease Control and Prevention. Guideline for hand hygiene in health-care settings: recommendations of the Healthcare Infection Control Practices Advisory Committee and the HICPAC/SHEA/APIC/IDSA Hand Hygiene Task Force. *MMWR Recomm Rep*. 2002;51(RR-16):1–45.

For More Information

ASHP statement on professionalism. *Am J Health Syst Pharm*. 2008;65(2):172–4.

Cantor J, Baum K. The limits of conscientious objection—may pharmacists refuse to fill prescriptions for emergency contraception? *N Eng J Med*. 2004;351(19):2008–12.

Manasse HR Jr. Public health: conscientious objection and the pharmacist. *Science*. 2005;308(5728):1558–9.

Ray M. Curbside conversation about noblesse oblige and moral commitment. *Am J Health Syst Pharm*. 2006;63(7):666–9.

Ross LF, Clayton EW. Religion, conscience, and controversial clinical practices. *N Eng J Med*. 2007;356(18):1889–92.

Rudd G. Healthcare without conscience—unconscionable! *Ann Pharmacother*. 2007;41(11):1903–5.

Weinstein BD. Do pharmacists have a right to refuse to fill prescriptions for abortifacient drugs? *Law Med Health Care*. 1992;20(3):220–3.

CHAPTER | 6

Understanding and Applying HIPAA

Some laws and regulations are designed to control practices. Others are enacted to protect, and still others to facilitate. The Health Insurance Portability and Accountability Act (HIPAA) is an example of all three purposes in one large piece of legislation.

HIPAA *controls* with whom private patient health information may be shared and under what circumstances. In this way, it also *protects* a patient's privacy by prohibiting the sharing of certain information with those who have no need to see it. But it is not so prohibitive that it discourages health care personnel from sharing important information when they do need it. In other words, HIPAA gives procedures to *transfer* medical information between institutions or offices that need it because they share responsibility for a patient's care.

What Is Private Health Information?

Let's look at what is considered private health information, or PHI. It includes a patient's demographic data, such as name, address, telephone number, age, ethnicity, religious preference, insurance, and even admitting diagnosis. To protect patients, HIPAA prohibits disclosing a list of the names of a health care provider's patients to anyone. In an outpatient setting, this regulation means pharmacy patients might be given numbers to notify them when their prescriptions are ready so that they don't have to be called by name. HIPAA also prohibits the posting of patients' names on a chart on the floor of a hospital where anyone walking by could read them.

Why Protect Health Information?

You might be thinking, "What's the big deal about mentioning a prescription as long as you don't say what it's for?" Or, "What difference does a list of names on a wall make, since

Protecting privacy extends to not talking about patients in the public areas of a pharmacy or hospital.

it's not mentioning embarrassing conditions?" Let's consider these situations.

In the example of calling out a name, suppose you have a child with a noncommunicable condition. Just as the pharmacist calls your child's name, the mother of a child who plays with yours walks into the pharmacy and hears that you are getting a prescription. Perhaps she concludes that your child has a serious condition, or she wants to know how your child is. What if the condition is something that might embarrass your child if word got out to other children?

In the second situation, a patient checks into the hospital for an uncomfortable test or procedure. A visitor walks by to see someone else, notices the patient's name on a posted list, and decides to drop in. For some this might be a nice surprise, but for others it is intrusive and interferes with rest and recovery. Furthermore, a patient in the hospital may not want to disclose a condition. This example illustrates why even basic demographic information must not be accessible to those who do not have a need to know.

Protection of information is considered so important that medical record numbers cannot be given out even if the names are removed. They are as sensitive as Social Security numbers. The inappropriate release of patients' medical record numbers can significantly violate their privacy, so these numbers should be used only for internal purposes—that is, within the system in which they are assigned.

Protecting privacy extends to not talking about patients in the public areas of a pharmacy or hospital. Voices carry. Stairwells, for example, can amplify a conversation—although nobody is close by, someone several floors below may be able to hear everything. A discussion about a patient in a cafeteria or local lunch spot might provide enough detail even without the name to allow neighboring diners to pick up information. Even if listeners incorrectly identify the patient being discussed, what they hear may lead them to the wrong conclusion about the similar case of a patient they do know. Perhaps they decide to share the erroneous information with the patient, giving false hope or inaccurate bad news. Can you imagine the patient's reaction to different information delivered by the treating physician?

Portability

Portability allows a patient's information to be shared by treating physicians and other health care providers. For example, someone from a hospital might call a pharmacy requesting the last dose or filling date of a medication a patient is supposed to continue receiving. This is a legitimate request, since hospitalized patients don't always have a list of medications with them. Patients might not be in a condition to answer questions about their medications, or they may give information about doses that differs from the usual treatment. For instance, a large normal man with no reason to be on a very low dose of warfarin might say that he is on 0.5 mg of the drug, but a call to the pharmacy determines that he is on 5 mg. Such a call maintains therapeutic dosing, preventing a potential iatrogenic, or treatment-related, condition.

Sometimes it is necessary to send entire charts. This should be done in a way that minimizes the chances of charts or information getting into the hands of unintended recipients. When information is given over the phone, reasonable care should be taken to ensure that the person is someone with whom it is appropriate to share the information. Assess how callers identify themselves and the type of institution from which they are calling. If someone seems questionable, it is prudent to verify the business, the caller, and the number through a reliable reference source. When medical records are sent electronically, they should be encoded in case they get delivered to the wrong recipients.

By providing for continuity of care between a patient's various health care providers, portability enhances the safety of health care delivery. When a primary care provider, a pharmacist, and others directly involved in a patient's care are able to talk with one another, potential problems are more likely to be avoided—for example, medical care that might be detrimental in certain situations is not given, or doses or medications that would be harmful given particular accompanying conditions are not prescribed.

Accessibility

Another provision of HIPAA concerns accessibility. Even though you *can* access records of people you know, you *may not* do so unless you are actively involved in their treatment or have a need to know. This privacy extends even to close relatives. A person does not have the right to access a spouse's medical records, nor can an adult child access a parent's chart without specific power of attorney. It does not matter if the child is a physician or pharmacist unless the person is actively treating the patient or has specific signed permission from the patient.

Need to Know outside the Realm of Health Care Delivery

Sometimes it is necessary for someone in the billing department to access records for billing purposes. An insurance company may want to know why a patient received a particular procedure or medication. For insurance purposes, most health care practices and facilities have patients sign waivers that allow sharing necessary information with insurance companies. Even so, information not directly related to a claim should not be disclosed. This might include procedures the patient has had that are unrelated to the condition or a psychiatric issue (e.g., depression) that has nothing to do with the current condition. And while a patient's weight might be helpful for dosing, it clearly doesn't relate to the bill.

Within a facility, "need to know" is specifically defined. If a third party is billed using diagnosis-related group (DRG) pricing, the diagnosis must be sent to the billing department but not necessarily the day-to-day procedures, physicians' notes, medications, or other information. Even within a department, if staff members don't have direct business related to a patient, they cannot ask about patient information. For example, suppose a celebrity is a patient at your pharmacy. At some point, he brings in a prescription that another technician fills. The order is already dispensed by the time you come in. The patient paid cash, so there are no billing issues. At this point, what the prescription was for, who prescribed it, the celebrity patient's address, and any other related information are none of your business, and snooping in the patient's records is a violation of HIPAA.

Accountability

The last important issue in understanding and applying HIPAA is accountability. In health care institutions, a record of who has had access to private health information needs to be kept. Even when it is appropriate for a health care provider or other employee to access PHI, a system to track who has obtained access to files is necessary.

Most organizations use computer databases to log who has had access to patients' PHI. Often, PHI is stored within the same computer systems. Each person who may have a need to know specific information or a need to access patients' files should have a unique log-in code. Access to files unnecessary for the performance of an individual's job should be restricted. Even where it is not possible to restrict access electronically, it is a violation to view a file of interest when there is no professional reason or to "surf" the files for a patient or file of personal interest.

It is the responsibility of each person to ensure that a personal log-in code is not shared intentionally or indirectly by leaving it exposed on a desk or workstation. On a shared computer, the user should always log off when finished working with PHI to prevent unauthorized access by others. Log-in codes must be carefully protected.

Access to files unnecessary for the performance of an individual's job should be restricted.

Summary

Health care is best delivered when there is a climate of trust between patients and their health care providers. HIPAA defines and regulates the use of patients' private health information. It allows for the sharing of information among those who need to know professionally and protects such information against inappropriate retrieval by those who have no need for it. By providing health care providers with the ability to share information with each other and take patients' full medical background into consideration, HIPAA helps ensure that patients receive the safest and most appropriate care.

ACTIVITY

Answer the following true-false questions. Discuss what makes the false ones false.

1. By definition, as long as people are licensed, they have a need to know PHI.

2. Information can be shared between two people treating the patient without the patient's consent.

3. Whenever someone calls for information and they have a release, you should give them everything in case they forgot to ask for something.

4. Portability means you should keep the charts thin enough to put in a regular-size envelope in case you have to send it somewhere.

5. Health information includes birth date.

6. HIPAA only applies to information that came into existence after it was implemented.

7. Business people in an organization never have a need to know as far as personal health care information is concerned.

8. PHI stands for public health information.

Answers: 1.F; 2.T; 3.F; 4.F; 5.T; 6.F; 7.F; 8.F

For More Information

Baker KR. The impact of HIPAA on pharmacy. *Ann Pharmacother.* 2003;37(10):1522–5.

Fitzgerald W Jr. *HIPAA Compliance Handbook for Community Pharmacy.* Alexandria, Va: National Community Pharmacists Association; 2003.

Mackowiak LR. Pharmacists and HIPAA. *Am J Health Syst Pharm.* 2003;60(5):431.

Office for Civil Rights. *Summary of the HIPAA Privacy Rule.* Washington, DC: U.S. Department of Health & Human Services. Accessed at www.hhs.gov/ocr/privacysummary.pdf, August 6, 2008.

CHAPTER | 7

Role of the Technician in Different Practice Settings

Certain skills are thought to be universally necessary for a technician to be successful. Although this is generally true, some settings require interpersonal skills or physical stamina more than others do. When you are looking for a good career match, it is wise to know the expectations in a particular practice site before choosing it. When you are managing people, matching their attributes with job requirements is one way to maximize talent and increase job success rates.

Physical skills are things we do with our bodies. Because technicians are usually in motion, stamina is important. The following physical skills are helpful:

▋ Extended standing (accommodations are available in some settings)
▋ Seeing
▋ Lifting
▋ Kneeling
▋ Bending
▋ Walking
▋ Reaching
▋ Pulling and pushing
▋ Hearing (accommodations are available in some settings)

Many of the skills needed for pharmacy technology can be learned. These skills include the following:

▋ Mathematical calculations
▋ Medication names
▋ Typing and computer skills
▋ Sterile technique
▋ Basic knowledge of the body, diseases, and treatments
▋ How to fill a prescription or an order

Some skills needed to be successful in pharmacy technology are related to personality and ability to communicate. These skills can be enhanced, but the basic traits should be inherent. Personality traits that make a successful technician include the following:

I Likes people
I Communicates well
I Empathetic
I Listens well
I Outgoing
I Friendly
I Helpful
I Well organized
I Good time manager
I Remembers people and faces
I Detail oriented

Let's look at the different practice settings and the skills that complement them.

ACTIVITY

List the skills you have that would make you a successful pharmacy technician. Put an asterisk next to your best attributes.

Community Pharmacy Practice

Community pharmacy is commonly known as retail pharmacy. While individually owned pharmacies may still be viable in smaller towns and communities, the traditional corner drugstore has given way to chains in larger communities. As the profession of pharmacy changes, however, new opportunities in the community are arising in medication therapy management. People who chose to work in this environment must like people and have a lot of compassion.

The role of the technician in a dispensing pharmacy is varied. Frequently, technicians are the faces of the pharmacy and the employees seen first and most often by patients. It is important that technicians present themselves in a professional manner. Technicians generally greet patients, receive their prescriptions, and record basic information, such as demographics, insurance, and allergies. Technicians may be instructed to obtain the pharmaceutical histories of patients, or this may be done by pharmacists. Technicians also refer patients directly to pharmacists if appropriate—for example, when patients request drug information or medication recommendations.

New opportunities in the community are arising in medication therapy management.

Once prescriptions and pertinent histories have been obtained from patients, technicians may type and fill the prescriptions, preparing them to be checked by pharmacists. Only pharmacists can make decisions about the appropriateness of particular prescriptions, and only pharmacists can dispense medications and counsel patients. Technicians, however, generally take care of the financial aspects. Technicians in retail settings also answer telephones, take refill requests, order and shelve inventory, maintain the appearance of the pharmacy, and take care of preauthorization requests and insurance claim adjudication.

As pharmacists become more involved in medication therapy management, technicians may work with them in a role similar to a nurse's aide. In this case, technicians may take patients' histories on a form, organize patient flow, and prepare the monitoring forms for pharmacists. These technicians are most likely responsible for handling insurance reimbursement or for securing payment directly from the patient.

Compounding Pharmacies

Some pharmacies specialize in compounding. The technicians in these settings are responsible for setting up the ingredients for compounds that are not commercially available. Compounding pharmacies may start with raw ingredients, or they may use a commercially available product and change its dosage form to something easier for the patient to use. Items compounded in these settings may be tablets, capsules, liquid dosage forms, topicals, and suppositories. Some compounding pharmacies also fill prescriptions for commercially available medications, but others do not. Unless a pharmacy is set up for sterile manufacturing and complies with all United States Pharmacopeia (USP) 797 requirements, it will not compound sterile products.

Technicians working in hospitals must be able to move rapidly from one task to another.

Technicians in compounding pharmacies may greet patients, receive prescriptions, type or generate labels, and do the bulk of the measuring, mixing, and packaging of medications under the direct supervision of pharmacists.

Hospital Settings

Hospitalized patients are generally acutely ill. Many have unstable conditions necessitating emergency attention because a delay may cause significant permanent harm. Most patients are hospitalized for a short period of time. Once they are stabilized or the procedures requiring close observation have been completed, they either return home or go to a facility offering a lower intensity or level of care, such as a skilled nursing facility.

Technicians working in hospitals must be able to move rapidly from one task to another if necessary. Although many of the responsibilities are similar to those of community pharmacy technicians, sometimes routine assignments must be delayed for "stat" orders that need to be addressed. Such flexibility is essential for people working in this type of environment.

Satellite and Dispensing Pharmacies

The role of technicians in the hospital setting is diverse. In the inpatient dispensing area, technicians are responsible for preparing orders for dispensing. They may process new orders, or they may fill a 24-hour supply of medication in what are generally called patient cassettes. Technicians determine what is needed for the patients by printing a 24-hour fill list or a medication administration summary, depending on the computer software used.

Most hospitals use a unit-dose system. This method of dose delivery involves dispensing as a unit the correct milligrams, milliliters, or tablets a nurse will need for a given dose. For instance, if a patient has an order for divalproex 750 mg taken three times a day, the technician prepares three doses of a 500-mg tablet that is attached in some way to a 250-mg tablet. If the patient is unable to swallow the tablets and requires the liquid equivalent, the dose is 15 mL. Since the product comes in a multidose bottle, the technician draws 15 mL into a single syringe for each dose, thus supplying the nurse with a prefilled syringe containing the correct dose. This method allows the nurse to easily double-check the patient's dose. By pre-measuring or preparing the dose, there is less room for error.

Inpatient technicians may pre-pack or prepare unit doses from bulk supplies when unit doses of products are unavailable commercially. When a rarely used medication is ordered and requires pre-packing, the technician usually prepares just a few doses for the specific patient. In cases of medications used for a broad range of patients, sufficient quantities to fill expected orders for weeks or months may be unit-dosed.

Once unit-dose cassettes have been filled and checked for accuracy, technicians exchange the cassettes. Newly filled cassettes are distributed to nursing stations, replacing cassettes distributed the day before. Items left in the cassettes are credited and monitored to determine if patients have been given all ordered doses.

Technicians working in these environments interact with hospital staff more than with patients. They need to be efficient, accurate, and flexible because order demands require shifting focus quickly.

Sterile Compounding

Inpatient technicians may also work in an area called sterile products or intravenous admixtures. Because such products are often injected directly into the vein, good technique ensures that no cores or glass particles from original containers are introduced into them. Should such objects be injected into the vein, they could cause fatal clots to form.

Sterile products are used to treat the sickest patients. Because these patients are frail and their immune systems are already compromised, care must be taken to make sure that bacteria and other organisms are not introduced into sterile products in the process of making them.

To help prevent infectious material from being put into sterile products, admixture areas used for compounding these items must comply with USP 797 guidelines. For example, positive pressure rooms are included in the guidelines. They provide a sterile area for compounding antibiotics, electrolyte replacements, hydrating solutions, eyedrops, and chemotherapeutic injections. Some hospitals also prepare total parenteral nutrition (TPN) admixtures.

Accuracy and concentration are particularly important when preparing sterile products.

Chemotherapy hoods and biological hoods are two types of technology that not only protect the product from the environment but also protect the compounder (i.e., the technician) from the product. These hoods have special ventilating systems that send air out of the room rather than at the technician, and they have protective glass separating the preparation area from the technician.

Besides good technique, accuracy and concentration are particularly important when preparing these products. For the most part, a clear liquid is introduced into another clear liquid. Thus, unlike solid dosage forms such as tablets and capsules, once two or more liquids are mixed, it is impossible to determine without expensive assays what is actually in a container. It is also impossible to remove the medication once it has been administered. Unlike topical agents, which can be washed off before being absorbed, or oral medications, which can be removed by stomach pumping or other means, once a product is administered parenterally, it is irretrievable. The only way to manage a problem is through supportive care and time.

To make working in sterile-product areas safe, technicians need to be especially good at calculations and especially alert so that mistakes are prevented. Technicians working in sterile-product areas have minimal interactions with other health care providers and patients, yet their job function is one of the most important to everyone involved.

Besides filling orders and cassettes and preparing sterile dosage forms, inpatient or hospital technicians may be responsible for inventory, stock supplies, telephones, greeting nurses who come to the window, and floor stock inspections. Floor stock inspections are monthly inspections of nursing stations to ensure that medications are properly and securely stored. During an inspection, pharmacy staff also make sure that expired products have been removed from the shelves and that any adulterated medications are not being stored.

Home Health Care Pharmacies

Home health care pharmacies specialize in long-term treatments that were traditionally administered in the hospital. These pharmacies and the technicians who work there fill orders for TPN, enteral nutrition, home intravenous therapy (home IVs), implantable pump medications, and some inhalation therapies. Sometimes patients are on a 6-week course of antibiotics for osteomyelitis, an infection of the bone. They aren't sick enough to require hospitalization, but they do need parenteral therapy. Other patients may require TPN for life.

Most of the preparation of products compounded in these pharmacies occurs in a sterile hood and frequently in a sterile room. Because of the large volume of each order, many facilities have huge vats in which TPNs and other products are manufactured. Unlike sterile-product pharmacies in hospitals, many of these pharmacies start with raw materials.

The customer base of home health care pharmacies centers around hospitals, skilled nursing facilities, and case managers. The institutions have their own home health care pharmacies, but in most hospitals, case managers or discharge planners refer patients to outside home health care pharmacies. Ultimately, the patient becomes the direct contact, but the initial introduction is usually made through another health care provider.

Public relations is a key element in the success of these pharmacies. In small operations, the proprietor (owner) or partner scouts for contacts and business. As these pharmacies expand their business, salespeople may be hired to contact potential referral sources. Technicians with outgoing personalities are likely candidates for such sales positions because they understand their operations and are able to answer questions from potential customers. They might also offer to speak at support groups for patients who require ongoing home health care, such as a cancer survivors group or a Crohn's disease group.

Besides manufacturing home health products, these pharmacies usually supply the durable medical equipment needed to use the medications. Examples of durable medical equipment are IV tubing that connects the medication to the patient, needles, bandages, "port" cleaning supplies, and medications to keep the port open. A port is the site of attachment to the patient. Technicians are usually responsible for assembling the supplies. After pharmacists check everything, technicians package the supplies for delivery or pickup.

Other functions of technicians working in these pharmacies might include scheduling routine manufacturing, scheduling deliveries, ordering everything from supplies to raw materials and medications, and billing insurance companies. Technicians might be assigned to call patients to make sure they will be home for their deliveries, confirm that they need supplies, or just check to make sure everything is OK. Technicians are also responsible for keeping sterile rooms clean and maintaining the general tidiness of the pharmacy. Technician managers might be responsible for making assignments to other technicians.

Mail-Order Pharmacies

Mail-order pharmacies are high-volume operations that primarily fill prescriptions to treat chronic diseases. These prescriptions are usually refills because while the mail-order pharmacy has the capacity for high-volume output, the prescriptions are usually filled at a distant location and then sent to patients or their local dispensing facility. For instance, in operations such as the Veterans Health Administration and the health care provider Kaiser Permanente, many of the medications filled by centralized or mail-order pharmacies are delivered to local operations for dispensing to patients as though the prescriptions were filled on-site. The time required to send something usually prohibits the use of mail-order pharmacies for initial prescription fills.

Mail-order pharmacy operations capitalize on volume filling by using expensive technology that is only cost effective when huge numbers of prescriptions are being filled. The use of technology reduces the number of personnel required, in turn lowering salary and benefit costs. However, the initial technology costs are difficult to recoup in small operations.

Using technology requires some mechanical competence and concentration. Technicians need to be aware of the levels of drugs in the filling sleeves because failure to load a machine at the proper time can significantly delay the operation. Loading the wrong drug into one of the sleeves affects hundreds of prescriptions, which then need to be pulled and redone. Imagine the impact this would have on a service that produces 70,000 prescriptions in an eight-hour shift!

Functions of technicians in these settings include routine maintenance and cleaning of the automated machines. In addition, technicians in these operations have functions that are similar to those in a retail setting. In mail-order pharmacies, technicians take refill requests off the refill request line, fill and set up prescriptions, order inventory and supplies, and prepare envelopes for mailing. Unlike technicians in retail settings, technicians in these practice settings have minimal contact with patients.

Using technology requires some mechanical competence and concentration.

Long-Term Care

Long-term care facilities are residential treatment centers for patients who cannot live in their own homes but do not require the acute care of a hospital. If patients have health care issues that require nursing services, they go to a skilled nursing facility, or SNF (pronounced "sniff"). Otherwise, they might go to an assisted living facility, where the needs of patients do not require the same high ratio of trained nurses to patients necessary in a skilled nursing facility. An assisted living facility provides care for chronic conditions and assistance with daily living requirements, such as bathing, dressing, and medication reminders.

Since patients in long-term care facilities have ongoing needs, medication is provided per patient in quantities similar to the number of days supplied to outpatients. However, many facilities require that the medication be bubble packed with the patient's name and that each dose be packaged in one bubble. Technicians working in pharmacies catering to long-term care facilities may find themselves bubble packing and preparing monthly or biweekly supplies of medication.

Because patients are provided for by the facilities, the proprietors or managers of the facilities are the pharmacies' customers. Marketing and salespeople might call on various long-term care facilities in the area for business. As with home health care, the sales and marketing end of long-term care might appeal to technicians who like meeting new people and developing relationships.

Personnel Recruitment Functions

Some chain pharmacies and temporary staffing agencies use technicians as personnel recruiters. A recruiter is someone who scouts for talent and invites potential employees to apply for a job. Frequently, recruiters work at professional seminars and pharmacy school job fairs, and they may make "cold calls" by phone or online.

Cold calling is a technique used by salespeople to solicit the interest of potential buyers or clients, who may not even think they are in the market. A pharmacy recruiter, for example, might call or e-mail a pharmacist or technician about a job that might be of interest if he or she were aware of it.

Recruiters engage people in initial conversation and pre-interview them. They have to understand the needs of the hiring firms, as well as the types of pharmacists and technicians who would be best suited for particular positions. Recruiters are scouting for talent—pharmacists and technicians—as much as they are selling the companies using their services to the interested talent. Often recruiters are evaluated on their ability to deliver applications, so they might also need to help potential employees fill out applications. Recruiters need to be able to enthusiastically discuss the benefits of working for their particular hiring companies while also being able to answer recruits' concerns and questions.

Other Practice Settings

Infusion Centers

Infusion centers are clinics where patients go to receive intravenous medications that require administration by a nurse. This type of clinic may be associated with a particular physician group, be part of a larger health care facility such as a hospital campus, or be a freestanding center. Items that are infused into outpatients in an infusion center may include chemotherapy, biological material such as intravenous immunoglobulin (IVIG) for immune deficiencies, and blood products. Technicians supporting pharmacists in these venues prepare the doses for patients in much the same way that technicians working in sterile-product areas of hospitals do. Unlike products prepared in home health care pharmacies, these products are prepared one patient at a time and one dose at a time.

In slower operations, technicians may get to meet the patients, but most often contact will be with nurses over the phone or when they pick up medications. Technicians in these facilities usually work in teams with three to four other technicians and pharmacists.

Pharmacies Associated with Investigational Drug Trials

Meticulous record keeping is important in every aspect of pharmacy, but it is particularly important in investigational drug trials. A drug investigation is a study designed to prove (or disprove) that a new entity is safe and effective in treating a particular ailment. The records related to a trial are the very documents the U.S. Food and Drug Administration (FDA) uses to approve a medication for distribution to the public.

Trials may also be designed and conducted to prove that one treatment is better than or as good as another. These trial results have broad implications for how different diseases are treated.

Working in an investigational pharmacy or a pharmacy that in part handles investigational products is similar to working in a retail setting or an inpatient facility in terms of labeling and preparing medications. There are additional steps, however, for technicians or pharmacists.

They need to make sure that each patient has signed an informed consent before any medication is dispensed. This is usually completed by the principal investigator and then forwarded to the pharmacy. Nonetheless, the pharmacy needs to make sure it has been signed.

Medication that is provided in cards containing individual doses on individual days might need to have the anticipated day of the dose written in the appropriate space on the medication card. In addition to the label normally affixed to prescriptions and required by state law, explicit instructions for how and when to take a dose may need to be typed.

Investigational studies have a lot of paperwork. The investigational product needs to be checked in. Frequently, paperwork must be returned to the source to verify receipt. There are inventory logs and dispensing logs to keep. The pharmacist or technician has to make sure that patients are coming in for medication within the parameters set up by the protocol for the study. If there are deviations from the protocol, approval needs to be obtained and documentation needs to be verified before additional product is dispensed. In some arenas, the job of getting approvals falls on the principal investigator, but the request might be initiated by the pharmacy staff.

In double-blind studies, the product may come coded. The code may be supplied on the initial visit for the duration of the trial, or it may be determined with each visit. Either way, it is important to keep accurate records on the forms set up by the sponsor or the principal investigator. It is also important to verify that the right code has been given to the right person—failing to do so may invalidate data and be costly.

In single-blind studies, the patients may be blinded but not the investigator. For some studies, the pharmacist and the technician may have to encapsulate product to make sure that bias in product is eliminated from the start. Some studies require that a log for each patient be kept, as well as master inventory logs.

Logs for studies do not end with recording what is being dispensed. Unused drug must be documented, so patients are generally asked to return unused product and packaging. The returns are recorded and become part of the data to verify what each patient actually took. After all, how can you say whether something worked if the patient took only half the expected doses?

Sponsored studies are studies funded by an outside source in contrast to those initiated by a clinic, hospital, or physician's office. Sponsored studies have monitoring visits—scheduled spot checks by the sponsor to make sure that the study is being conducted appropriately. During these visits, records kept by the pharmacy are reviewed by the monitor for accuracy, legibility, and completeness. When a drug approval from FDA is awaiting the outcome of a study, a lot of money and promise rests on the results, so details are particularly important. In addition to meeting with a study monitor, a technician or pharmacist may meet with a company-sponsored auditor in expectation of an FDA audit or with an FDA monitor to verify that the study was conducted in an appropriate manner.

Drug Information

Some third-party payers and hospitals have their own pharmacy libraries and fact-finding pharmacists. In larger facilities, the efforts of these pharmacists may be supported by technicians. Technicians in drug information sites may be responsible for filing resources, answering phones or message machines, typing responses, and retrieving resources, as well as organizing the area and maintaining supplies. They may need to record callers' questions and their fields of specialty. This type of job might best be described as a combination of librarian and secretary.

As in most settings, knowledge of medications and diseases is necessary to ensure that messages and questions are accurately recorded. Technicians working in drug information areas need good receptionist skills, good organizational skills, good writing skills, and a high degree of professionalism, since they interact primarily with physicians, pharmacists, nurses, and other health care providers.

Technicians working at PBMs may be the first-line personnel to evaluate a treatment authorization request.

Pharmacy Benefits Manager Companies

Pharmacy benefits managers, or PBMs, are companies that manage pharmacy insurance for large employers. Examples of PBMs are Health Net, Medco, and Kaiser Permanente as its own PBM. These businesses try to control the costs of providing insured employees with prescription coverage by limiting the products paid for by the insurance. They contract with pharmacy manufacturers to get a particular rate for an agent or a rebate based on market share of a line of products. Bulk-purchase contracts lower costs by promising to purchase a specified minimum (large) quantity over a specified period. Market-share contracts usually specify what percentage of total purchases of the contracted items will be bought from the designated line. For instance, a PBM might have a contract stipulating that if 75% of antihypertensive agents are from a particular pharmaceutical manufacturer, then the PBM will receive the antilipidemic at a good price, or it may agree to additional discounts on the total purchases from that manufacturer. To meet these contractual agreements, PBMs have formularies to promote the preferred items and, frequently, penalize providers or patients or both for prescribed and dispensed items that are not on the formularies. Penalties to providers are in the form of reduced profit share, and penalties to patients may be in the form of higher co-pays.

Technicians working at PBMs may be the first-line personnel to evaluate a treatment authorization request, or TAR, for a nonformulary item. By PBM policy, some items may be routinely approved. The PBM provides technicians with a list of universally approved items. Technicians might simply be required to log the call in order for the plan to monitor expensive medications or nonformulary usage of these items.

Summary

Technicians work in many different areas. The choices made at the beginning of a career may be based on factors or interests that can change over time. Skill sets can be adapted to ease into another area of interest or completely changed during the course of a career. Understanding the different types of technician functions and settings helps a manager mentor employees. It also allows a manager to match work needs and assignments with the personnel who fit best.

ACTIVITIES

1. Identify an area of work that most interests you. Write an essay about why you think you would like working in that area.

2. Visit a pharmacy that does the kind of work that interests you. Interview the employees about their job functions.

3. Look for advertisements for technician jobs in your local paper or online. Inventory the skills being requested (e.g., second language or the years or type of experience requested).

4. Inventory your interests and attributes. Match them with the description of the type of pharmacy in which you would like to practice.

For More Information

ASHP long-range vision for the pharmacy work force in hospitals and health systems: ensuring the best use of medicines in hospitals and health systems. *Am J Health Syst Pharm.* 2007;64(12):1320–30.

Desselle SP, Holmes ER. Structural model of certified pharmacy technicians' job satisfaction. *J Am Pharm Assoc.* 2007;47(1):58–72.

Ivey MF. Re-engineering for dramatic improvement in the medication-use process. *Am J Health Syst Pharm.* 1995;52(23):2681–5.

Keresztes JM. Role of pharmacy technicians in the development of clinical pharmacy. *Ann Pharmacother.* 2006;40(11):2015–9.

Kreling DH, Doucette WR, Mott DA, et al. Community pharmacists' work environments: evidence from the 2004 National Pharmacist Workforce Study. *J Am Pharm Assoc.* 2006;46(3):331–9.

McAllister DK, Rittenback DA. Staffing pharmacies to meet the demands of patient-oriented care. *Am J Hosp Pharm.* 1994;51(24):3024–5.

Morris AM, Schneider PJ, Pedersen CA, et al. National survey of quality assurance activities for pharmacy-compounded sterile preparations. *Am J Health Syst Pharm.* 2003;60(24):2567–76.

Muenzen PM, Corrigan MM, Smith MA, et al. Updating the pharmacy technician certification examination: a practice analysis study. *J Am Pharm Assoc.* 2006;46(1):e1–6.

CHAPTER | 8

Third-Party Issues

Third-party payers—with the exception of the governmental third-party payers Medicaid and Medicare—are in the health care business to make money. Insurance companies are for-profit businesses. Fortunately, one of the ways they profit is by purchasing bulk health care services, making the cost to treat someone less than it is when services are purchased for one person at a time. This is no different than buying a product such as toilet paper in bulk rather than in individual packages.

Another way insurance companies make money is by having many healthy people pay into the same pot of money as sick people do. This practice spreads the health care costs among users and nonusers of services while providing nonusers with coverage in case they become users. Over the years, many well people felt the need to get back some of the money they paid in insurance premiums and obtained care that they marginally needed. To discourage unnecessary or excess use of insurance benefits, co-payments and other fees for services—albeit at reduced rates from the total costs—have been instituted in addition to insurance premiums.

Share of Costs

The share of costs is the portion of payment that the user, or patient, pays for the health care provider's services. In the case of pharmacy, it may be for the product or for a medication management visit. In the case of office visits or hospitalization, it is usually a fee for services from the health care provider, such as medical care, laboratory tests, surgery, or a room.

The share of costs may be a deductible that needs to be met before the third party pays for any services, or it may be a fee assessed for each visit to a health care provider. A deductible is a set amount of money the patient must pay up front for any services before the insurance company starts to pay. The total deductible can be met with one expensive

The share of costs is the portion of payment that the user, or patient, pays for the health care provider's services.

treatment or a combination of many services. Deductibles provide a way for insurance companies to lower premiums by having patients pay for most "usual" costs. Deductibles can range from being fairly small amounts (e.g., $500) to being rather large (e.g., $2,500).

A share of costs in the form of a co-pay means that the patient pays for part of every service. This arrangement may have a higher premium because it ensures that even the least costly service is billed in part to the insurance company. It also means that patients share a financial burden for each use of the health care system. Sometimes this helps defer any inappropriate or frivolous use, which helps reduce overall costs.

It is most important to fill out any paperwork or enter the record of payment into the electronic system as soon as possible. Especially in the case of deductibles, patients usually cannot access their insurance coverage until the deductible has been met and paid. A delay in confirming payment may delay or inhibit access to further health care. Delays in submitting electronic third-party claims requiring a deductible may affect future care as well. Such cases include medications that require specific time intervals to elapse before refills can be dispensed.

Medicare prescription coverage combines the co-payment and deductible types of insurance plans. It is commonly referred to as Medicare Part D. Under this program, insurance is initially available to everyone—all users have access to a certain amount of coverage up to a particular point. Depending on the plan, there may or may not be a co-pay. After a certain dollar amount has been reached, patients have a window of no coverage, known as the "donut hole." Once a specified amount of out-of-pocket expenses has been incurred, patients can begin receiving additional financial benefits, which often include a larger share of the total cost than what the insurance paid before the donut hole.

Since most pharmacy bills are paid at least in part by third parties such as insurance companies and since the third parties aren't present at the time of the transactions, it is necessary to correspond with them. This is now done almost exclusively as online claims adjudication. In most systems, patient accounts are created in a computer database. Then, each patient can be linked with the insurance company's information when the account is set up in the pharmacy's computer system.

Before we look at the details of third-party adjudication, let's clarify a few insurance terms and issues.

Formularies

A formulary is a list of medications that are available to patients through an insurance plan or a health care organization. Most insurance companies have a formulary that defines what medications they will pay for and in what quantities. Hospitals and other agencies may have a formulary as well to reduce inventory and storage costs.

The decision to include particular medications on a formulary is usually made by a committee with input from prescribers, pharmacists, and other health care workers who will use the medications to treat their patients. Formularies often have at least one representative item from each therapeutic class of agents to treat most maladies.

The decision about which representative medication is placed on the formulary is sometimes financially based. For instance, an insurance company or a hospital may choose to have one particular agent in a therapeutic class over a similar product simply because of the relative costs of the two. The relative cost may be based on the manufacturer's average wholesale price (AWP), a mathematical formula, or a contract where a price is determined by taking into account a guaranteed market share. That is, the hospital or insurance company entering into the contract promises a certain percentage of particular business to the manufacturer in exchange for a better overall price. Sometimes the decision to include one product over another is simply based on dosing schedule, with a once-a-day product generally considered more favorable for patients than an agent that requires more frequent dosing.

Formularies may be used to create tiered pricing plans. In some insurance companies, these determine the patient's co-pay. Since generic products are generally less expensive than brand-name products, there might be a $5 co-payment for a generic product and a $20 co-payment for the brand-name version. There may also be a preferred agent, but in the interest of providing for patients for whom the preferred agent doesn't work as well, alternatives in the same class may be available but with a higher co-pay.

An incorrectly submitted form will be rejected and may then cause a delay in getting an answer back for the patient.

Formularies can also include restricted medications. In the outpatient setting, such restrictions might have laboratory parameters—a requirement that a monitored lab value such as white blood cell count or glucose level fall within a particular range. For instance, filgrastim is an expensive inducer of white blood cells, so a formulary might restrict its use to patients whose white blood cell count is below a certain level. In other cases, a medication might be restricted to patients with certain ailments—for example, limiting the use of erythropoietin to patients with chronic renal failure or patients on dialysis.

In hospital settings, some restrictions are based on the service, or specialty. The use of expensive or certain broad-spectrum antibiotics might be restricted to infectious-disease physicians so that other physicians do not overuse the antibiotics. Inappropriate use or overuse of antibiotics renders them prematurely ineffective against the target bacteria, which develop resistance. In the case of the heart medication nesiritide, many hospitals restricted it to the cardiology service when it came out. They did not want other physicians to inappropriately use this expensive specialized treatment with patients who weren't suffering from severe congestive heart failure. In the pharmacy, personnel must be familiar with the restrictions so that clearances can be obtained when appropriate and drug treatments that are not optimal for particular patients are not inadvertently started.

Treatment Authorization Requests

Insurance companies have parameters for how often claims for the same item can be made, for what quantities are allowed, and sometimes even for what conditions certain medications can be prescribed. Sometimes, though, exceptions need to be made. For these instances, a treatment authorization request, or TAR, must be submitted (Figure 8-1).

Third parties are particular about the forms that are used to submit these requests. They are also strict about how these forms need to be filled out. An incorrectly submitted form will be rejected and may then cause a delay in getting an answer back for the patient.

For all claims, demographic information has to be complete. It is important when completing these forms that the

FIGURE 8-1

Example of a Treatment Authorization Request

CONFIDENTIAL PATIENT INFORMATION
TREATMENT AUTHORIZATION REQUEST

TAR CONTROL NUMBER
A119117875

NOTE: AUTHORIZATION DOES NOT GUARANTEE PAYMENT. PAYMENT IS SUBJECT TO THE PATIENT'S ELIGIBILITY. BE SURE THE PATIENT'S ELIGIBILITY IS CURRENT BEFORE RENDERING SERVICE.

Adapted from Medi-Cal Treatment Authorization Request form, California Department of Health Care Services.

Consult directly with the prescriber for the diagnosis and justification for the noncovered medication.

initial claim has the correct patient information, as well as the primary insured's information. If the patient is a dependent or spouse, not the primary insured, both the primary insured's and patient's Social Security numbers, insurance card numbers, and dates of birth may be needed. Make sure that this information is entered on initial enrollment into the pharmacy system and that it is updated regularly.

Along with demographics, the medication, dose, frequency of dosing, and reason for the prescription are essential to communicate to the third party. Do not guess at a diagnosis. Some insurance companies do not pay for off-label use of items. Also, do not record a diagnosis that the patient doesn't have, since this will become part of the permanent record and may make obtaining insurance in the future difficult—the "false" diagnosis will then be a pre-existing condition. To have the most accurate information on the claim, consult directly with the prescriber for the diagnosis and justification for the noncovered medication. The prescriber should also provide the alternative formulary items that were tried but were unsuccessful.

TARs require a justification explaining why the patient needs a medication not normally covered by the insurance company (Figure 8-2). "The physician wants it" is not a justification. A typical justification might be that the patient failed to respond to the medications normally used for the condition, followed by a list of what was tried and did not work. Other justifications might be that the patient is on a medication that is contraindicated with the usual treatment; the patient is allergic to the typical agents covered; or the patient has an orphan disease requiring a treatment that is not on the formulary because few people have the condition and the drug is expensive. By keeping expensive medications as nonformulary items, insurance companies make sure they are not paying for unapproved uses.

Cyclosporine is an example of a nonformulary agent commonly used for one condition. The treatment of choice for transplant patients, it is also an expensive, third-line agent for psoriasis. To help discourage random treatment of usual cases with third-line agents, Medicaid requires a TAR for cyclosporine in some states. Such petitions are universally granted for transplant recipients and often denied for all other purposes.

FIGURE 8-2

Example of a Diagnosis and Medical Justification on a Treatment Authorization Request

CONFIDENTIAL PATIENT INFORMATION
TREATMENT AUTHORIZATION REQUEST

FOR PROVIDER USE

TYPE OF SERVICE REQUESTED — DRUG OTHER
REQUEST IS RETROACTIVE? — YES NO
IS PATIENT MEDICARE ELIGIBLE? — YES NO
PROVIDER PHONE NO. ( )
PATIENT'S AUTHORIZED REPRESENTATIVE (IF ANY), ENTER NAME AND ADDRESS:

PROVIDER NAME AND ADDRESS:
PROVIDER NUMBER

FOR OFFICE USE
PROVIDER: YOUR REQUEST IS:
APPROVED AS REQUESTED   DENIED   DEFERRED
APPROVED AS MODIFIED (ITEMS MARKED BELOW AS AUTHORIZED MAY BE CLAIMED)
BY

NAME AND ADDRESS OF PATIENT
PATIENT NAME (LAST, FIRST, M.I.)
PATIENT IDENTIFICATION NO.
STREET ADDRESS
SEX   AGE   DATE OF BIRTH
CITY, STATE, ZIP CODE
PHONE NUMBER ( )
PATIENT STATUS: HOME   BOARD & CARE   SNF / ICF   ACUTE HOSPITAL

INSURANCE CONSULTANT
I.D.#   DATE
REVIEW COMMENTS INDICATOR

DIAGNOSIS DESCRIPTION:
Cachexia as side effect of AIDs
MEDICAL JUSTIFICATION:
pt needs surgery, has no appetite.
Needs to gain 10% body wt. prior to
procedure.

ICD-9-CM DIAGNOSIS CODE

COMMENTS/EXPLANATION

LINE NO.	AUTHORIZED YES	NO	APPROVED UNITS	SPECIFIC SERVICES REQUESTED	UNITS OF SERVICE	NDC/UPC OR PROCEDURE CODE	QUANTITY	CHARGES
1	☐	☐	☐	*Marinol 5mg*	3	0051-0022-21	60	$
2	☐	☐	☐					$
3	☐	☐	☐					$
4	☐	☐	☐					$
5	☐	☐	☐					$
6	☐	☐	☐					$

TO THE BEST OF MY KNOWLEDGE, THE ABOVE INFORMATION IS TRUE, ACCURATE AND COMPLETE AND THE REQUESTED SERVICES ARE MEDICALLY INDICATED AND NECESSARY TO THE HEALTH OF THE PATIENT.

SIGNATURE OF PHYSICIAN OR PROVIDER   TITLE   DATE

AUTHORIZATION IS VALID FOR SERVICES PROVIDED
FROM DATE   TO DATE
TAR CONTROL NUMBER
A119117875

NOTE: AUTHORIZATION DOES NOT GUARANTEE PAYMENT. PAYMENT IS SUBJECT TO THE PATIENT'S ELIGIBILITY. BE SURE THE PATIENT'S ELIGIBILITY IS CURRENT BEFORE RENDERING SERVICE.

Claims Adjudication

Most pharmacies have online claims adjudication. This type of communication allows for almost instantaneous transmission of a transaction. In turn, the pharmacy gets a response from the insurance company about whether the claim will be processed. If the claim is not going to be paid, the electronic response explains why the claim was rejected. Although the intent is to receive an instant response, sometimes errors occur at the time of the transaction and follow-up may be required.

For instance, a number of years ago, a pharmacist submitted a transaction for fluconazole 150 mg, the treatment of choice for vaginitis, albeit a relatively new standard of practice at the time. The prescription had been filled with three 50-mg tablets of fluconazole because that was what the pharmacy stocked. The claim was rejected. After calling to ask what the current approved agent was, the pharmacist was told by the third-party technician that it was fluconazole 150 mg. Upon further investigation, the pharmacist discovered that the insurance company paid based on National Drug Code (NDC) number, not on actual intent. Although it would pay for one tablet of fluconazole 150 mg, it would not pay for three fluconazole 50 mg. Such arbitrary electronic transaction requirements make for lengthy processing of what should be routine claims. In this case, a lot of work went into getting approval to dispense the correct dose to the patient and get paid for it.

Large-volume organizations have several personnel devoted to claims adjudication. They might be technicians or a combination of technicians, billing assistants, and even accountants. They authorize payment, do bookkeeping, perform audits, and help pharmacists and other health care personnel with formulary management.

Summary

Claims adjudication is a communication between the pharmacy and the insurance company. The bulk of the work is handled by technicians and nonpharmacists. Most claims are handled electronically. Timely submission of claims helps the pharmacy with monetary flow and helps the patient by keeping track of the patient's co-payments and deductibles in a timely manner.

ACTIVITIES

1. Look up the formulary of an insurance company online. How is the medication list arranged? Are alternative treatments listed next to one another?

2. Fill out the TAR form on page 113 with you as the patient. You will be requesting pregabalin for diabetic neuropathy. You have already tried amitriptyline and gabapentin, but they both made you too sleepy during the day.

For More Information

De Natale ML. Understanding the Medicare Part D prescription program: partnerships for beneficiaries and health care professionals. *Policy Polit Nurs Pract*. 2007;8(3):170–81.

Depue R, Stubbings J. Medicare Part D: selected issues for plan sponsors, pharmacists, and beneficiaries in 2008. *J Manag Care Pharm*. 2008;14(1):50–60.

Goldman DP, Joyce GF, Zheng Y. Prescription drug cost sharing: associations with medication and medical utilization and spending and health. *JAMA*. 2007;298(1): 61–9.

Kilian J, Stubbings J. Medicare Part D: selected issues for pharmacists and beneficiaries in 2007. *J Manag Care Pharm*. 2007;13(1):59–65.

Madden JM, Graves AJ, Zhang F, et al. Cost-related medication nonadherence and spending on basic needs following implementation of Medicare Part D. *JAMA*. 2008;299(16):1922–8.

Medicare program; Medicare prescription drug benefit; final rule. *Federal Register*. 2005;70(18):4193–4585.

Medicare Web site: www.Medicare.gov.

Mullins CD, Palumbo FB, Saba M. Formulary tier placement for commonly prescribed branded drugs: benchmarking and creation of a preferred placement index. *Am J Manag Care*. 2007;13(6 pt 2):377–84.

CHAPTER | 9

Maintaining Medication and Inventory Control Systems

Effective management of medications and other inventory involves much more than replenishing existing stock. The development of systems that ensure an adequate supply of medications to conduct business efficiently—that is, to fill orders and prescriptions—requires planning, implementation, and flexibility. Besides reordering product, technicians in charge of inventory control must review packing slips and invoices for accuracy, regularly inspect stock to determine appropriateness for current business, predict the impact of shortages and of U.S. Food and Drug Administration (FDA) and manufacturer product recalls, make necessary changes to keep up with prescribing trends, regularly inspect shelves and stock to remove outdated and soon-to-expire medications, and return eligible medications for credit before the window of opportunity closes. Systems must be user friendly for the pharmacy staff who will be making requests, using the product, and tracking usage. Also, the financial feasibility of the plan needs to be kept in mind. Table 9-1 summarizes the elements of inventory control.

TABLE 9-1
Inventory Control

Basic inventory control involves:
■ Ordering stock
■ Rotating stock
■ Determining stock quantities
■ Shelving orders
■ Pulling outdated stock
■ Returning recalled medication

Deciding Appropriate Stock Levels

Most pharmacies enjoy daily service delivery from their wholesalers. This allows pharmacies to have less money tied up in inventory. It also ensures that most pharmacies can fill a prescription within 24 hours of receiving it. Nonetheless, certain essential medications must be stocked regardless of how many patients may require them, and a working supply of "fast movers" is also vital.

Fast movers are the most frequently prescribed medications a pharmacy sees. They can vary depending on a pharmacy's location and clientele. For instance, if the pharmacy is associated with or close to a large cancer treatment facility, it might stock larger quantities of oral chemotherapeutic agents, antinauseants, narcotic pain medications, and corticosteroids than would be found in the usual community pharmacy. Student health facilities and pharmacies in areas with many young or single people dispense more birth control and antibiotics relative to the number of diabetic agents and heart medications than the typical pharmacy does. In a pharmacy where a known patient has a rare disease, a supply of the drugs for the patient's condition is appropriate. Such agents would not be kept on hand in many other pharmacies, because of the infrequent occurrence of the condition.

The pharmacy technician responsible for ordering has to decide with the pharmacy manager what the appropriate levels of medications are for that pharmacy and how many times a year they would like to "turn over" the stock. Turnover refers to the times the investment in inventory will be "respent" in a time period. For instance, if the inventory is worth $100,000, will the total order for medications be $100,000 per quarter, per month, or per two weeks? Turnover reflects sales volume, but not every medication is dispensed in the designated period. Fast movers account for the difference between 100% turnover of the entire inventory and 100% financial turnover.

The amount of inventory to carry and the selection of what to carry in that inventory are determined by many variables. The most important is what a store can reasonably afford in terms of a financial investment that allows it to be able to immediately fill most of its first-time prescriptions and prescriptions for waiting patients. Although a pharmacy can request that current patients call ahead for refills to ensure that an item is in stock, it is harder to capture new business if patients cannot get prescriptions filled promptly and without having to come back. Inventory is also affected by a store's sales volume or the number of patients in a facility's beds (the daily census). For example, a 100-prescription-a-day store carries less inventory than a store in a much busier area, and more stock has to be available if a facility is running at 95% capacity versus 50% capacity.

The ease of obtaining particular agents as well as generic availability may affect how much stock is kept on hand. When a shortage of a drug occurs, many pharmacies that normally carry a two-week supply might order enough to cover several months. A shortage from one manufacturer of a multisource drug creates less of a hardship than a shortage of a single-source, heavily prescribed agent.

Routine Ordering

The person in charge of inventory control should set up a system to keep track of what needs to be ordered. In some pharmacies, the system is a simple replacement strategy—if you used it, reorder the amount needed to replace what you used. Sometimes the plan is "if you used it up, reorder" or "if there isn't enough to fill another prescription of the usual quantity, reorder." Some pharmacies use a par-level system—a pre-determined minimum quantity is kept in stock at all times. For instance, if the quantity on hand should be four bottles of 100 and two and a half bottles are used in a day, then three bottles are ordered for the next delivery. Other pharmacies create a list on which needs are written down by filling pharmacists and technicians and ordered at the end of the day by the ordering technician. The list can include requests from patients, anticipated needs generated by a pharmacist, and replacements of what has been used from normal stock to fill prescriptions during the course of the business day. Smaller operations may have a box where used containers are tossed, and at the end of the day, the ordering technician punches in the order from the "stash of trash" (containers). Finally, computer interface systems can generate orders on the basis of what inventory has been ordered by physicians (in inpatient settings) or filled as prescriptions (in outpatient settings). Except in the case of an interface system, an order

Make sure that the order has been delivered in good condition and that all the billed items have been received.

has to be manually entered into a system or, at the very least, transmitted from a scanning device to the wholesaler.

Checking in an Order

It is important to make sure that the order has been delivered in good condition and that all the billed items have been received. When an order arrives, a spot check to make sure it is not too hot and does not appear damaged is appropriate. Before the order is placed on the shelves, it should be checked against the packing slip or invoice to ensure that everything has been received. Most wholesalers provide stickers with each item's cost and inventory number. The stickers should be placed on the items before they go on the shelves. The information they provide helps save time in reordering. These tags also allow staff to more easily assess use, since the date received is often included.

Storage Requirements

Laws require that medication dispensed to a patient be unadulterated and in good condition. Maintaining temperature and climate control and monitoring expiration dates are ways to ensure that medication is dispensed in good condition.

While it could arguably be said that the temperature is too hot for medication when the staff is uncomfortable, the United States Pharmacopeia (USP) range for room temperature is between 59°F (15°C) and 86°F (30°C). The range for refrigeration is between 36°F (2.2°C) and 45°F (7.2°C), and freezing is below 32°F (0°C). Some agents, however, have different storage requirements. The temperature range may be narrower than that defined by USP, or the storage temperature before dispensing may be different from the temperature that is acceptable when the patient is using the item. For instance, insulin should be stored in a refrigerator to maximize its shelf life, but it can be stored for 28 days at room temperature. Therefore, if the patient is going to use the supply in less than a month, refrigeration after dispensing is not necessary.

All package inserts include the storage requirements (Figure 9-1). Storage information is usually the last item on the insert. In addition, items that require refrigeration usually have a notice on the outside of the box or carton. The

FIGURE 9-1

Storage Requirements on a Package Insert

> **Store at 20° to 25°C (68° to 77°F). [See USP for Controlled Room Temperature.]**
>
> **Protect from light.**
>
> Dispense in a tight, light-resistant container as defined in the USP using a child-resistant closure.
>
> **PHARMACIST:** Dispense a Medication Guide with each prescription.

packaging of frozen items also states that they must be kept at a temperature below freezing. These items should arrive at the pharmacy in appropriate containers that maintain the required temperature.

Items that require constant refrigeration or freezing temperature usually arrive in insulated containers marked as such. The medications are packed with ice bricks or dry ice. Some medications that have a longer shelf life when refrigerated, such as insulin, may come from the wholesaler in the general delivery. Therefore, it is important to read all packaging information before putting an order away to make sure that an item that arrived unrefrigerated does not require refrigeration for the long term. Once you are familiar with the products, you will learn where most go and only have to check the unfamiliar ones.

The package insert also notes whether a medication is sensitive to moisture, usually presented as "store in a tightly closed container." If a product is light sensitive, the package advises to "store away from light." Most medications come in opaque containers, eliminating the problem of defining their climate requirements for pharmacy stock. But once you repackage a medication for a patient's prescription, how do you control moisture and exposure to direct light?

For repackaging, most pharmacies only stock child-resistant amber vials and bottles. Most inpatient facilities that blister pack or pre-pack medications in unit-dose packages use amber bubbles. By using the most stringent packaging for everything, pharmacies save money in inventory and storage costs associated with having both clear and amber containers.

Child-resistant caps meet the air-tight requirement of medications that should not be exposed to moisture. Pharmacists generally counsel patients not to keep medication in bathrooms where moisture varies because of showers. In inpatient or long-term-care facilities, showers are not an issue.

If you are responsible for inventory control, it is important to keep up with ordering vials, bottles, needles, syringes, labels, and other items necessary for running the business of the pharmacy.

Stock Rotation and Regular Maintenance

Stock rotation and inventory control minimize unnecessary expenses for any business. Stock rotation means that the newer products with longer expiration dates are not used until the older items of the same product have been dispensed. Usually this is done by moving existing inventory to the front of a shelf and placing items from the recent shipment in back. The "first in, first out" rule helps reduce waste in the form of unusable product expiring on the shelf.

Expiration dates are required on all medications and many devices whether they are over the counter or prescription. Because pharmacies have to stock some medications that are not used often, routine checks of inventory for outdated material is recommended. Inpatient facilities do this once a month in all nursing and pharmacy storage areas as part of the Joint Commission requirements. It is a good idea to go through the inventory once a month in other settings. Even with prudent stock rotation, items can go out of date without being noticed—for example, when a patient on a rarely prescribed medication changes medication. With frequent monitoring, staff can remove slow movers before they expire and return them to the wholesaler for credit while they are still usable.

Returns and Recalls

Careful monitoring of inventory flow enables the technician to predict when stock will become outdated before it is used. Some drugs have short expiration dates. Other times, outdating occurs because drugs fall out of favor, such as when a new product becomes a more preferred agent for a particular condition. Drug potency may also expire when a regular patient with an uncommon regimen leaves the area. Or, a patient may change regimens or stop using the pharmacy.

By monitoring stock, the technician is often alerted to excessive stock relative to use, allowing for timely returns to the wholesaler. Such prudent return of in-date inventory enables the pharmacy to get credit because the wholesaler can still use the product. Crediting medication rather than disposing of expired drugs stretches inventory dollars and maximizes profit.

To get credit for medication, the technician must check with the wholesaler about policy and protocol. Some whole-salers have parameters for how long before an expiration date a medication must be returned in order to receive full or partial credit. Wholesalers may have specific forms or steps that must be taken before credit is issued, so it is important to be familiar with their terms and conditions.

FDA mandates drug recalls when products do not measure up to the standards specified. FDA, however, does not initiate all recalls. Manufacturers may also send them. Pharmacies are commonly notified of these through alerts that are delivered with an incoming order from the wholesaler or through the mail. Sometimes a mailed notification is sent both to individual pharmacists and to all licensed pharmacies.

Recalls are classified as I, II, or III, depending on how serious the harm to the public might be if the agent weren't immediately removed from the shelf. In a Class I recall, the product poses a potentially serious threat to public health if it continues to be dispensed. Class III may be a small labeling error on a product that otherwise meets safety criteria. Class II recalls fall in between the other two categories in terms of the effect on health and the use of the product.

Upon receiving a recall, it is important to follow the rec-ommendations in the letter. Generally, recalls are lot specific instead of involving the entire supply of the agent. Most often, only unused stock needs to be removed from the shelf and returned to the manufacturer. In these cases, previously dis-pensed product does not have to be recovered, so patients who were possibly administered or dispensed a recalled prod-uct do not have to be notified. It is a rare case that requires notifying patients who might have already received or taken a product and who may have some medication remaining.

Careful monitoring of inventory flow enables the technician to predict when stock will become out-dated before it is used.

Once a recalled item is removed from the shelf, follow the directions for obtaining credit or replacement stock.

Narcotics and Other Controlled Substances

Narcotics have special regulations that require closer monitoring and special order forms. In some states, they also require special forms to dispense. To be certified to stock and dispense narcotics, or more appropriately "controlled substances," a pharmacy must have a DEA number, issued by the U.S. Drug Enforcement Administration. Individual or business DEA numbers are also assigned to wholesalers from which pharmacies receive controlled substances and to prescribers who may prescribe these agents. Invalid DEA numbers and people using suspended DEA numbers should immediately be reported to authorities.

Controlled substances include narcotics and agents with high abuse potential and high addiction potential. High abuse means that the agents may be diverted from their medical use to recreational purposes or other unsanctioned uses. Addiction potential refers to the tendency a particular agent has to cause the body to "require" its use because without it, uncomfortable or life-threatening withdrawal symptoms may occur. In the strict sense of the term, narcotics are agents derived from or similar to opium. Other agents that are controlled substances include benzodiazepines, stimulants, and many sedatives and hypnotics not of the benzodiazepine family.

There are five classes of controlled substances. Class I controlled substances are those with no medical justification, such as ecstasy, heroin, and marijuana. Class II substances are heavily abused opioids, stimulants, and barbiturate hypnotics. Class III substances are primarily opioids in combination with over-the-counter pain relievers, such as acetaminophen or aspirin, and anabolic steroids, such as testosterone. Class IV substances are mostly benzodiazepines, and Class V substances are mostly cough suppressant combinations and diphenoxylate/atropine. The higher the number of the class of drugs, the lower is its abuse potential.

Inventory control is important for all controlled substances and most stringent for Class II narcotics. These items must be ordered on a triplicate form—DEA 222—issued by the U.S. Department of Justice. Two copies of the form are sent to the supplier, and one copy is kept in the pharmacy. The supplier sends the second copy to DEA upon filling the order. There cannot be cross-outs on the DEA 222 form. Further, it must be signed by the pharmacist-in-charge or that person's designee each time an order is made. This must be done in addition to the ordering done online or by scanned information.

The exact inventory of Class II drugs must be available at all times. Most pharmacies do this by keeping a running inventory. Each time a Class II prescription is filled, the amount used is subtracted from the inventory log and the remaining stock is verified. These logs are kept in both inpatient and outpatient settings. In a hospital setting, running inventories are also kept at each nursing station, and complete inventories are done at each change of shift. Some pharmacies perform an inventory of all Class II medications monthly whether or not they have been dispensed. Regardless of what kinds of inventories an operation chooses to perform, a biannual inventory of all controlled substances is mandated and needs to be recorded and sent to DEA.

A biannual inventory of all controlled substances is mandated and needs to be recorded and sent to DEA.

Summary

Keeping track of inventory and knowing what to order in a pharmacy is a complex process that requires planning, careful record keeping, and flexibility. Besides planning for the most common prescription needs, the astute manager is able to predict seasonal trends and plan for shortages. The high cost of some drugs necessitates being familiar with the needs of the pharmacy's patients in order to streamline inventory while being able to accommodate patients and keep expenses to a minimum.

ACTIVITIES

1. Visit pharmacies in several different practice settings to find out how their inventory is controlled.

2. Using the information from your research, evaluate the systems you would use.

For More Information

Hoffman JM, Shah ND, Vermeulen LC, et al. Projecting future drug expenditures—2008. *Am J Health Syst Pharm*. 2008;65(3):234–53.

Holt RT, Larson DS, Scheil ES. Assessment of formulary development in a small hospital. *Hosp Pharm*. 1988;23(7):649–52, 656, 666.

Hsu EB, Casani JA, Romanosky A, et al. Critical assessment of statewide hospital pharmaceutical surge capabilities for chemical, biological, radiological, nuclear, and explosive incidents. *Prehosp Disaster Med*. 2007;22(3):214–8.

Lin AC, Huang YC, Punches G, et al. Effect of a robotic prescription-filling system on pharmacy staff activities and prescription-filling time. *Am J Health Syst Pharm*. 2007;64(17):1832–9.

Salamie D. Modern inventory analysis techniques. *Am J Health Syst Pharm*. 2000;57(4):351–67.

Skibinski KA, White BA, Lin LI, et al. Effects of technological interventions on the safety of a medication-use system. *Am J Health Syst Pharm*. 2007;64(1):90–6.

Smolarek RT, Powell MF, Solomon DK, et al. Pharmaceutical perpetual inventory: a comprehensive approach. *Top Hosp Pharm Manage*. 1988;8(2):59–65.

Wilson S. Inventory management to reduce costs: a case study. *Hosp Pharm*. 1995;30(9):759–61, 765–6.

CHAPTER | 10

Workflow Management

Workflow management is creating systems that maximize productivity. It takes personnel numbers and talents into consideration when tasks are assigned. At the same time, systems must be set up within the physical layout to produce a logical, stepwise flow of work that minimizes backtracking and excess movement. Good workflow systems plan for the norm while allowing for flexibility when staffing or work volume fluctuates. Poor workflow designs can reduce the efficiency of an operation and weaken the staff's morale. Table 10-1 provides questions to consider in designing a good workflow.

Let's look at several examples where a system may have been conceptually appropriate but fell short in the execution. Let's also explore issues that need to be considered so that the questions in Table 10-1 can be adequately addressed.

TABLE 10-1

Designing a Good Workflow

- Has space been designed to maximize efficiency for reduced or expanded workloads?
- Are telephones and computers reasonably spaced and sufficient in number to facilitate workflow, not interrupt it?
- Have unnecessary steps in procedures been eliminated?
- Does the order of the steps in the process make sense?
- Is excessive movement by personnel necessary to carry out the work?
- Are materials and medications close to the workstations where they are needed?
- Is a system in place to handle electronic breakdowns? Short staffing?

Good work-flow systems plan for the norm while allowing for flexibility when staffing or work volume fluctuates.

Oversystematizing

Example 1

In a retail pharmacy, prescriptions were separated into three groups: waiters, pick up today, and pick up later. The waiters were prescriptions dropped off by people who intended to wait for them to be filled. Pick-up-today prescriptions were either refills called in or prescriptions dropped off. Patients came to the pharmacy later in the day to get them. Pick-up-later prescriptions were those that patients said they would call for on a subsequent day.

All prescriptions that came into the pharmacy were typed by a single technician. This person prioritized the typing on the basis of when the medications were to be dispensed to the patients. The typed labels with the original prescriptions were then sent by conveyor belt to the pharmacists and technicians filling the prescriptions. At this step, the prescriptions were actually shuffled again into the various piles.

Since the pharmacy was busy most days, the waiters were continually accumulating during normal business hours. What happens to the rest of the prescriptions in this setup? What happens if the same-day pickups are not integrated into the workflow of waiters? Can you imagine how many hours of staff time are wasted in a week separating all the prescriptions into different piles?

Example 2

To alleviate the problems inherent in systems such as the one described in example 1, another pharmacy divided the workflow into categories of prescriptions. One team worked on prescriptions for patients undergoing procedures, one on waiters in the pharmacy, one on refills, and so forth. As it happened, the distribution of work was not even. Although the walk-in business was particularly busy Monday through Thursday, postprocedure patients were light in the beginning of the week but much heavier toward Friday and right before a big holiday. In addition, when the pharmacy opened, refills were a large part of the business. With mail-order pharmacies becoming the preferred providers for many prescription plans, refill business dropped significantly.

What personnel issues might arise from such a distribution of work? How do you reassign staff to accommodate different workloads? How could a manager build a system so that staff members interact as a single pharmacy team rather than work in teams divided by function?

Example 3

In another pharmacy, the sterile-product hoods were divided into the TPN, or total parenteral nutrition, hood (because of a mixing machine that facilitated the preparation of TPN), the "regular" hood, and the chemotherapy hood (because of the special biological protection needed in the hood design). Because the products took different amounts of time to prepare and the complexity of their preparation varied, some technicians completed their work well before others.

As in the previous example, what incentives could be used to motivate technicians not to spread the work out and use more time than necessary? Should pharmacy maintenance tasks such as ordering, sterility testing, and stocking be assigned by taking into account the difference in time to accomplish primary tasks? Should there be a mechanism in place to share "prep" work needed to complete assignments that are more labor intensive than others?

What about round-the-clock operations? Many hospitals have skeleton staffing on the overnight, or "graveyard," shift. These shifts are usually less busy by volume, but the orders are for patients who are most critically ill. Such orders are often the most time-consuming to process. Do regular maintenance assignments given to the midnight shift take into account a busy night? Is there an inherent and understood expectation that maintenance activities are to be attended to during downtimes?

In these three examples of oversystematizing, unnecessary functions were created. In the first, a sorting function evolved. Instead of focusing on the prescriptions, a staff member also worked at dividing the work. In the second and third examples, the work was allocated in such a way as to discourage flow of staff between functions during slow or busy times.

The examples illustrate the need to have a design with flexibility. With too much structure, employees are not apt to break out of their assignments. With too little structure, every task becomes someone else's responsibility. Rotating assignments allows for cross-training and maintenance of skill sets and provides the manager with resources to interchange staff between job functions. In addition, it gives team members variety in their job functions, which promotes fresh ideas and develops empathy for one another's challenges. All things being equal, routine assignments may work for certain staff members who prefer consistency in their work as long as such a division of assignments does not give the impression of favoritism or unearned benefit.

Physical Impediments to Maximizing Workflow

In the design of a viable workflow, it is important to consider the physical layout as well as staffing options. The design of a pharmacy should take into account high-use items and make these items easily accessible to those who need them. For instance, even if drawers on the side hold every size vial needed for a week, it is inefficient to have each technician or pharmacist walk over to them for every prescription that is filled. Likewise, syringes and needles must be within reach from a hood in a sterile manufacturing area, and frequently used medications need to be near the dispensing area, even if it means storing them out of alphabetical or some other order. Too frequently, the amount of walking required to get from one part of an operation to another wastes time.

Example 4

Let's look at a pharmacy designed to accommodate 600 to 1,000 prescriptions a day. With that many prescriptions, it is easy to have lots of personnel close to every area of the pharmacy. This particular pharmacy had a multiwindow reception area, and each station had a computer for entering demographics and prescriptions. The typists fed the typed prescriptions through a window behind them, placing the prescriptions on a conveyor belt to be transported to the line of pharmacists and technicians filling them. Once filled, the prescriptions were sent through a window at the end of the assembly line to the dispensing pharmacists.

Sounds reasonable, right? The problem was that in the beginning, the pharmacy was filling fewer than 35 prescriptions a day. With such low volume, the operation could only afford one pharmacist. In most cases, one pharmacist would be adequate for that volume, but the layout was not flexible enough to work efficiently with only one person. The assembly-line wall was more than 18 feet long. The window behind the reception area with the computers was not close enough to the stock to allow the filling operation to be run from there. The dispensing windows were not furnished with computers to allow data entry at that point. As a result, the sole practitioner was sprinting all day long. The take-home message: pharmacies with large amounts of space need to be designed to accommodate varying volume and staff size. A similarly designed pharmacy solved the problem by cutting an adaptable walkway reasonably spaced along the length of a counter. An adaptable walkway is a countertop that can be lifted to pass through and can be left down when additional counter space is needed.

Pharmacies with large amounts of space need to be designed to accommodate varying volume and staff size.

ACTIVITY

Think of ways to design an efficient workflow in the type of operation you would like to manage.

Centralized and Decentralized Stock

The accessibility of supplies is a central issue in managing workflow. In sterile manufacturing areas, proximity of parenteral bags, needles, syringes, and medications to the hoods is important. When a gowned person has to go in and out of the hood area repeatedly, the cleanliness and sterility of the hood becomes questionable. Keeping needles next to syringes makes sense, since they are used together. Stocking for hood areas individually also makes sense, since the use of the various items is high for each hood. Such a supply reduces both unnecessary movement and downtime for preparation. Backup supplies for restocking, however, may be kept in a central area for all hoods to share.

Alphabetizing stock by generic name is standard in most pharmacies. In some cases, however, keeping emergency medications near the pharmacist dispensing them saves critical time in an emergency. If an operation has a high

When you look at workflow, it is important to think about not only the physical aspects but also the sequence in which tasks are done.

enough volume of pediatric patients to support a team for filling those orders, pediatric medications may be arranged in a dedicated area. Other specialty items may also be stored out of the area where routine medications are kept. Such items may include topical ointments and creams, inhalation devices, ophthalmic preparations, radiology contrasts, and anesthetics. Determining the best setup for the pharmacy is facilitated by observing the operation for a period of time to see how things are working.

Often, a new manager taking over an existing operation finds that the physical space has already been designed. When this is the case, improving efficiency is still possible with minimal expense and without knocking down walls. Small portable storage bins may be helpful for setting up movable stock to create a second or third fast-mover section. Reallocating functions that are not part of a multiperson production team to an area off to the side may enhance the flow of work between people working on the same tasks.

Order of Tasks

Many operations have the technician as the first line of access for order processing. This may not be appropriate, however, from the standpoint of efficiently taking care of the pharmaceutical evaluation of orders.

In a retail or clinic setting, a workflow where a technician receives the prescription, types the label, and then has the order reviewed by a pharmacist may free the pharmacist from answering questions such as, "In what aisle is the toilet paper?" It does not, however, promote good pharmaceutical care. It may take 15 to 20 minutes or more before a pharmacist sees the order, and by that time, if a problem is detected, the patient may have waited unnecessarily. Reviewing a prescription for completeness, appropriateness, contraindications, or insurance problems before starting on it is a good first step. Therefore, personnel best suited to perform such a review should be in a position to do so.

The same holds true for the workflow in a hospital setting—for example, when the technician prepares an order before a pharmacist evaluates the patient's kidney function, age, and other medications. If all items are billed before they are administered, it's likely that there will be a lot of time spent issuing refunds for medication that was refused or discontinued before administration.

So when you look at workflow, it is important to think about not only the physical aspects but also the sequence in which tasks are done in order to eliminate unnecessary delays, waits, and time spent undoing work.

Issues Especially Relevant to Retail Settings

In high-volume outpatient pharmacies, there are basically two ways to run the workflow. One is to have a technician-and-pharmacist team work the same prescriptions from start to finish—that is, the person receiving the prescription is the same one or part of the same team that dispenses it. The other way is an assembly-line approach in which each member of the team has specific functions, but the whole operation works as one unit. Most operations use an assembly-line operation. Either is workable, though, depending on the physical layout and the clientele.

Where the work is divided in an assembly line is arbitrary and depends on the operation. Sometimes it makes sense to have one set of people take prescriptions in and prepare the labels and another set fill and dispense. Other times, intake, typing, filling, and dispensing are done by separate teams. In such a case, clear written communication of any unusual information to tell the patient needs to be attached to the order so that the dispensing pharmacist can easily find it, understand it, and communicate the information to the patient. Still other times, one team may follow the process from start to finish.

Even with these functions accounted for, time and personnel need to be allocated for refill processing, including taking requests from the phone or phone tree, answering the phone, taking verbal prescriptions, and ensuring adequate inventory. One way to reduce the impact of refill business on unscheduled work is to promise refills the next day or two days later. This should be done on the message machine to reduce the volume of unnecessary calls. Still, the work needs to be integrated into the workflow.

Make sure that you have accommo- dated the time and prescription needs of each patient to the best of your pharmacy's ability.

Planned and Unplanned Work

Let's look at a few ways to accommodate the different types of work rather than the personnel doing the work. If the staff works only on new prescriptions for patients who are in the waiting area, a large backup could develop. It's important not to overly delay filling items for patients who are not currently waiting at the pharmacy or else all prescriptions become wait- ers. The purpose of asking patients to plan ahead and call in orders for refills is to avoid having them wait and to reduce the amount of unscheduled rush work. If the pharmacy can determine when most patients call in orders or which days are busiest, staffing and other assignments can be planned. Planned work needs to be incorporated into the daily work- flow of unplanned work.

Some pharmacies do two or three waiters for each refill so that the waiting patients don't have too long a wait and the planners—the people who called in—also aren't incon- venienced. Larger pharmacies may rotate staff to areas where they only do refills. In multishift operations, slower shifts do the refills. It doesn't matter who does them as long as they get done quickly and efficiently.

Each refill should be reviewed within 24 hours of receipt so that needed supplies can be ordered and received in a timely manner. When the pharmacy is out of a medication or does not have a full supply of a medication, patients should be called as soon as possible to allow them to make new plans. Such plans may include rearranging a schedule to pick up the prescription on a different day or coming in for part of the supply.

Large, Bulky, or Cumbersome Orders

One other type of prescription set that causes work to back up is the large order. Suppose you have several orders of one or two prescriptions each and then a patient shows up with 13 prescriptions. Obviously, this order takes longer to complete than the small orders do. Think about the following questions and how each choice might affect potential business:

▌ Should you make this patient wait until all the other orders are filled? Consider that perhaps the person relies on some- one else for transportation.

▪ Should you fill all the prescriptions in the order received? People in line behind the patient with the large order would then have a long wait. How many times do you want to answer the question, "How long does it take to put pills in a bottle?"

▪ Should you ask the patient if he or she could come back at a specified time or the next day to avoid a lengthy wait in the pharmacy? This would allow you to process the other prescriptions in a timely manner and not cause everyone to wait an excessively long time.

▪ Should you tell everyone behind the patient that the wait will be particularly lengthy? By communicating the waiting time, people can plan how to spend their time.

How do you find the right answers to these questions? You need to make sure that you have accommodated the time and prescription needs of each patient to the best of your pharmacy's ability and that you have communicated this information. The answers will vary with individual patients. Some will volunteer to return at a later time. Some will want to be taken care of in a timely manner during the visit. Some returning patients will present you with a long list of refills that they want while they wait. While you can work with all patients to request advance notice for refills, keep in mind that the pharmacy is operating to serve the patients, not vice versa. Somehow you have to accommodate everyone.

ACTIVITY

When workflow is affected by a large order, how can you get each waiting patient's cooperation? Practice wording your explanation and request with others.

Hospital and Long-Term Care Issues

In an inpatient area, the concepts are similar, but the clientele is different. Patients in a hospital do not have options for where to get their medications. However, they are usually not the people showing up at the pharmacy window. Most often the people coming to the pharmacy are nurses who need doses for patients. Preparing new orders promptly is important for good working relationships and for patient care, but it is also mandated by regulating agencies. It is essential that routine and regular checks for new orders occur during all shifts. Fortunately, in most hospitals the orders are computer generated and printed directly in the pharmacy. In rare cases, they are sent via pneumatic tubes or handwritten. The pharmacy staff or some other designee then needs to regularly check nursing stations for these orders.

Technology has also evolved so that supply is readily available at nursing stations in automated dispensing machines. The pharmacy is responsible for the release of the medication in a timely manner, which is usually done by a pharmacist verifying an order electronically. This allows access to the automated dispenser by the nurse for the particular patient. Another related pharmacy issue is to ensure adequate stock is available in the automated dispenser. A technician is usually assigned this task.

What about other daily or scheduled orders? How do they get done? Most pharmacies designate staff to fill cassettes. With automated dispensing units, cassette filling time is substantially reduced from the days when everything needed to be placed in individual cassettes. Nonetheless, to be most efficient and to reduce the number of changed orders that need to be processed, arrangements to change cassettes for a 24-hour period should be made so as to capture the largest number of changes that will occur during hours when medications are given. For instance, let's say that the most frequent dose is four times a day—one dose is given first thing in the morning, one around lunchtime, one around dinnertime, and one at bedtime. Most physicians make rounds in the morning, so most changes are done by early afternoon. Such planning gives about three hours in the late afternoon to update the cassettes with any changes and to deliver the cassettes to the nursing stations before the late afternoon and early evening doses are needed.

Sometimes, the staff available is insufficient to allow for such distribution or filling. Perhaps all the cassettes can be filled with the routine medication by early afternoon, but there is not enough late-day staff to change and deliver cassettes in the late afternoon. If this happens, the operations manager needs to be aware that there may be more updating and nurse visits for such units. It also means that the nursing stations with early delivery should be the ones with more stable patients or the ones closest to the pharmacy so that the nurses don't have to be away from their units longer than necessary.

Problems Delay the Workflow in Any Area

Regardless of the practice setting or the nature of the workflow, problems arise that hamper the filling of orders or prescriptions. Should each team "own" the problems it uncovers, or should there be a special problem-solving team? Is it more efficient to have designated problem solvers, or might the time it takes to communicate the problem to another person take longer than solving it on your own? Should guidelines be established addressing when to refer a problem to someone else and when not to? Note that staff members should not ask for help simply to avoid doing work they find cumbersome.

Planning Trips Saves Time

Optimizing steps saves time. Even in an operation where an individual is responsible for completing the whole order or prescription—as opposed to the assembly-line approach—there will be times when one person can run errands for everyone. For instance, a storage room may be located away from the pharmacy. Before going to that area, the person should check if anyone else needs something from there. Also, there may be situations where it makes sense for only one person to make all deliveries rather than have everyone out of the pharmacy at once.

Saving Steps: Building Efficiency into the Physical Layout

In one operation, the pharmacy designer took into account the obvious notion that accessing drugs on the shelves is done to fill prescription orders. Instead of setting up the operation so that a stock bottle was removed from the shelf, brought to a centralized filling area, used, and reshelved, the designer included small work surfaces amid the shelves. This reduced the retracing of steps to replace a stock bottle.

In the in-patient setting, steps can be saved by arranging stock so that items with a common use are placed together.

The technician filling the prescription set it up at the filling station closest to the place of origin of the stock bottle and brought the finished order to a centralized area for checking. Naturally, this only works if there is a printout of what the product looks like for the pharmacist to check.

In the inpatient setting, steps can be saved by arranging stock so that items with a common use are placed together. For hospitals with a large pediatric practice, the pediatric medications can be arranged together, and likewise, other specialty items should be close to one another. Critical-care items or supplies commonly requested by nurses but not available in the automated systems should be near the dispensing window to provide easy access and minimize retrieval time. If the area is particularly large, the design might also include surface areas on which a technician prepares doses.

Space management is also necessary in pharmacy benefit management offices and billing operations. Arranging the area for keeping resources, references, and personnel who can answer questions near staff who need them saves walking and phone time.

Table 10-2 summarizes some points to consider in designing a good workflow.

TABLE 10-2

Tips for Devising Good Workflows

- Workflow has to be manageable with large and small staffs if flexible staffing exists.
- Rigid job assignments box staff in.
- Proximity of staff to supplies reduces unproductive time and motion.
- Maintenance activities need to be part of the workflow without interfering with good patient care.
- Be mindful of the average reasonable time to perform a task.
- Be willing to take into account reasonable additional time needed for emergencies and equipment failures.
- Account for staffing highs and lows.
- Test workflow systems for a reasonable period of time before redesigning them.
- Combine errands to reduce staff downtime.
- Use technology to reduce unnecessary movement or steps.

Prioritizing

Part of workflow strategy involves prioritizing several high-priority items at once. Think about the following situations.

Situation 1: How Does Rank Count?

A nurse comes to the window needing a medication for a code blue. At the same time, another nurse shows up for a stat dose of clonidine, a fast-acting agent that lowers blood pressure. Then, a supervising nurse shows up for a stat laxative. Meanwhile, a doctor calls to request formulary information. Think about the following questions:

▌ Whom should you address first?
▌ Are all stat orders really stat?
▌ Does the rank of the employee affect the immediacy of the request? That is, is a doctor more important than a nurse or a respiratory therapist? Is the patient's condition the most important variable?
▌ How do you evaluate the order of importance of the requests?

Situation 2: How Does Timing Play a Role in Prioritizing?

It has been a very busy day. It is 4:30 pm. The medication order needs to be put into the system in the next 30 minutes or else the pharmacy will not have an order delivered tomorrow. A longtime patient came into the pharmacy 10 minutes ago with five new prescriptions. The patient is not feeling well and wants to go home. You also know that one of the crabbiest patients will be at the pharmacy in 45 minutes, and his prescription isn't ready either. The pharmacy is short one technician for the later shift. Everyone is working hard. Think about the following questions:

▌ Should the patients or the medication order come first?
▌ What do you think would happen if the pharmacy's order didn't get transmitted? How might this affect patient care?
▌ Of the two patients, which one should get priority?

Sometimes the right answer one day will be different from the right answer another day.

Situation 3: How Does the Severity of a Situation Affect Prioritizing?

You are working in an inpatient satellite pharmacy. The pharmacist is busy verifying orders, and it is your job to set up the medications from the verified orders. It is also your job to answer the needs of nurses at the window and to answer the phone when more than one line rings at once. You have orders for a heart attack patient in the emergency room, a new mother in labor and delivery, and a patient on the general medicine floor who needs a maintenance dose of an antihypertensive. You also have an order for a stat pain medication from the nurse at the window. Just then the phone rings. Think about the following questions:

▌ Which should you take care of first?
▌ When should you answer the phone?
▌ Is a heart attack more important than pain?

ACTIVITY

For the three situations about prioritizing, think about your answers and discuss them with colleagues.

General Rules for Prioritizing

Prioritizing is something we all do every day. There will be times when it appears that there is no right answer. In fact, in some of the previous situations, there are shades of gray. Sometimes the right answer one day will be different from the right answer another day. For instance, in the situation where it is late in the day and the order has yet to be placed, there are two responses, depending on the circumstances. First, if nothing in the order is particularly needed for a prescription or order the next day, then you might skip a day and place the order when things quiet down, knowing that it will be delivered one day late. It may also be possible to call the wholesaler to see if a late order could be accepted. Second, if the order contains medications needed to fill prescriptions the next day, then ordering is a high priority.

As far as patients are concerned, the rule of thumb is first come, first served except when waiting would have immediate health consequences for a patient. Health consequences include increased or prolonged pain, a gastrointestinal emergency, or an acute asthma attack. They generally do not include inconvenience, although pharmacy visits should be as convenient as possible for the patient or the nurse.

ACTIVITY

Think about the following:

■ As a manager, how will you convey your priorities to your staff?
■ How do you teach staff members to recognize priorities? To know when it is appropriate to ask for help?
■ Is functioning as a team member teachable?

Summary

Workflow management is a multifaceted part of a manager's responsibilities. The design of an operation should consider form and function, the size of the staff, and the changing volume of work. To minimize wasted space and movement, people and resources need to be brought close together. Staff members need to be educated in how to decide when they need to ask for help and how to prioritize according to the goals of the organization. They also should be empowered to make decisions to facilitate the flow of planned and unplanned work. The manager must continually evaluate the system's successes and flaws. A good manager is able to recognize short-term occurrences (e.g., a two-week lull during the graduation of one set of residents and the initiation of the new ones, or a holiday rush) and long-term operational changes (e.g., the signing of a new contract or the loss of an existing one).

For More Information

Angelo LB, Christensen DB, Ferreri SP. Impact of community pharmacy automation on workflow, workload, and patient interaction. *J Am Pharm Assoc.* 2005;45(2):138–44.

Angelo LB, Ferreri SP. Assessment of workflow redesign in community pharmacy. *J Am Pharm Assoc.* 2005;45(2):145–60.

Ivey MF. Re-engineering for dramatic improvement in the medication-use process. *Am J Health Syst Pharm.* 1995;52(23):2681–5.

McAllister JC III. Collaborating with re-engineering consultants: maintaining resources for the future. *Am J Health Syst Pharm.* 1995;52(23):2676–80.

Skrepnek GH, Armstrong EP, Malone DC, et al. Workload and availability of technology in metropolitan community pharmacies. *J Am Pharm Assoc.* 2006;46(2):154–60.

CHAPTER | 11

Staff Management

Many managers feel that personnel issues are the most challenging part of their jobs. Personnel concerns range from whom to hire to whom to retain when downsizing and everything in between, including evaluating, motivating, and disciplining staff and distributing assignments fairly and equitably. In addition, sometimes a manager has to resolve interpersonal conflicts.

Hiring staff is one of the most important managerial functions. Sometimes managers acquire staff because they are hired into situations where the staff is in place, such as when a previous manager retires or leaves. Other times, staff attrition gives managers the opportunity to make hiring decisions.

Coming into a situation where you are replacing a manager can be difficult. If you moved up the organizational ladder, there may be resentments among those with whom you previously worked because you were chosen over someone else. These resentments may even come from co-workers who didn't want the job. If you come from outside the department, these same resentments can occur. You may also be compared with the former manager, which may or may not be advantageous.

If you are new to an organization, you need to assess the ambiance of the work area. One common rule of thumb advises that a manager wait about six months before making any major changes in an organization unless not doing so would be catastrophic. Very little in business is catastrophic.

One reason for waiting is that people in an organization react differently to the new player, the manager. Some are solicitous and unduly helpful. Others stand back and wait to see. Still others may try to sabotage existing rules or change policies that you may not yet have enough background on to make an informed decision. While anyone can be on good behavior for a short time, it takes months to assess who is a charmer and who is a legitimate worker.

Hiring should never be done without a careful review process. For a number of reasons, a great person on paper may not fit into a particular organization. Unless there is a long-range plan to completely restaff an area, it is important to consider how each hire fits into the current team. Just as a baseball team with a great pitching staff usually passes on an available great pitcher if it needs a third baseman, it is important for any organization to pass on a talented candidate who duplicates present skills when it needs someone with other assets. Thus, before you begin the interview process, it's important to evaluate the talents you already have on board so that you can choose someone with complementary attributes. It also means being aware of issues you may have in your staff that may require tempering.

For instance, suppose your existing staff is bored but functional. You might want to bring on someone with vim and vigor to inspire increased output or creativity. However, bringing an over-the-top cheerleader type into an unenthusiastic group set in their ways usually ends up with the newcomer being run out. Therefore, someone who can meet the old guard in the middle or has an interest that aligns the person with an older employee is a better fit than someone with an entirely different personality.

Interviewing to Hire

Interviewing should not be done hastily. It takes 30 minutes to more than an hour to assess a person for even the simplest task. Moreover, anyone can be on good behavior for a short time. Maintaining rapport is more difficult.

It also takes time to uncover a well-padded résumé or CV and validate an accurate one. Sometimes people make it appear that they were more directly involved with a program than they actually were. For example, for a vague résumé item like "health care fair," you might find out that the applicant worked a shift as part of the normal workday. Or, suppose a résumé notes that the applicant had been a consultant to a major news network. Your questions might reveal that on one occasion the applicant answered a phone call about a particular formulation from somebody affiliated with the network. One short, unpaid conversation does not make a person a consultant.

Probing questions about a résumé help separate good candidates from the bad ones. Nonetheless, some questions are illegal. They include questions about a person's age, marital history, religion, sexual preference, and health, unless health directly relates to one's ability to perform the job. Questions that are legal to ask can reveal areas of expertise, areas of concern, personality, and interests. Keep in mind that applicants can rehearse answers to standard interview questions. Broad, unusual questions can uncover much about personality and experience. Table 11-1 provides some examples of typical and creative questions.

A legendary figure in pharmacy had a poster in his office of birds in rows. All the birds looked alike except for one bird in one of the center rows. When interviewing potential employees, this director would often point to the poster and ask, "Where do you fit on my organizational chart?" With this question, he could evaluate many attributes of a candidate, including motivation, aspiration, goals, ability to think quickly, creativity, and individuality. Years later, even people who didn't get a job with him remembered the interview.

TABLE 11-1

Sample Interview Questions

Typical Questions	Creative Questions
What do you like about pharmacy technology?	Describe your ideal job position.
Where do you see yourself in five [or ten] years?	What is the most important contribution you've made to your current practice site?
Tell me about yourself.	What do you expect from a boss?
What do you like to do with your free time?	What is it about your hobby that makes it so exciting for you?
What do you want from a job?	What contributions have you made to your previous work sites? How will those experiences help you here?
What are your strongest attributes?	If you were in my position, what three attributes would you be looking for in a candidate?

It is the policy of many organizations to confirm only whether people were employed by the business and whether they are eligible for rehire.

The purpose of an interview is to gather enough information to be able to assess a candidate's capabilities and interest in the job. At the same time, a fair view of your organization should be given to ensure that the interviewee makes an appropriate choice as well.

References

References are part of a normal background check. With current business policies on providing references, it is difficult to get helpful information, so your interviews may be the best assessment of how well qualified applicants are and how well they would fit into your organization.

It is the policy of many organizations to confirm only whether people were employed by the business and whether they are eligible for rehire. Other personal references might provide better feedback. Having specific questions rather than just calling and asking if the person was a good employee may result in more useful information. You might ask, "Would you consider this person a team player?" or "How would you describe this person's job performance?" Other questions might include, "How was this person's attendance record?" or "How does this person work on a team?" Even if you ask good questions, a reference may not be willing or able by policy to answer them.

Often, people who worked for or with you ask if they can use you as a reference. You may have to follow a company policy that limits the type of information you can provide. If you are no longer working together or for the particular company, you may answer the questions as you see fit. Most often, someone seeking a reference regards you favorably. Those you agree to be references for—and those you ask to be your references—should be people you are comfortable saying positive and true things about.

Letters of recommendation are also sometimes questionable as a resource for information about candidates. They are often written from a template. Such a letter should not carry as much weight as a more personalized one.

The best letters point out particular behaviors. Usually these are favorable, but because particular actions are mentioned, you can decide how important they are to the operation. You should also look for omissions in the letter. If many important aspects of the job are mentioned but one is not, is it because the letter was getting too long or because the candidate has a major flaw in that area?

There are several things to think about when writing letters of recommendation. When someone approaches you to write a letter, be honest. Knowing that it is hard for a person to ask, you should agree to write one if you can. If writing the letter would be a hardship or if you cannot comfortably give a good recommendation, then you could suggest that you might not be the best person to write a letter. You could also suggest that someone who has known the person for a longer period of time would be a better reference.

When you write a recommendation letter, both the person's future and your reputation are at stake. Compromising your words to advance the person's career is not necessary. Sometimes, though, you can bend a bit. You could mention the person's attributes without comment. For instance, "Mr. Parker is a reliable employee." *Reliable* could mean that you could count on him to do his job or just that you could count on him to show up. Don't say a person is a fast learner when you know that it took him two weeks longer than everyone else to meet expectations.

The most effective letters tell the prospective employer what to expect from the person in a positive way. For instance, let's say you have an employee who has been with the company for 5 years. She is frequently 5 to 10 minutes late but outproduces everyone else once she arrives. In addition, when her assigned tasks are done, she volunteers to do other projects. Figure 11-1 shows one way you might write about her work in a letter of recommendation. Figure

FIGURE 11-1
Sample Recommendation

Jane Duncan has exemplary productivity. She consistently fills more prescriptions than any of our other employees. She regularly volunteers for additional tasks and often fills in the stock vials before their absence impedes our workflow. Another illustration of her self-motivation is our successful adopt-a-family project that she initiated and implemented for the holidays. Jane is also very pleasant with our patients. If you have any further questions, please feel free to call me.

11-2 provides another approach that addresses the issue of her late arrival in a positive manner.

FIGURE 11-2

Sample Recommendation

Jane Duncan has exemplary productivity. She consistently fills more prescriptions than any of our other employees. She regularly volunteers for additional tasks and often fills in the stock vials before their absence impedes our workflow. Another illustration of her self-motivation is our successful adopt-a-family project that she initiated and implemented for the holidays. Jane is also very pleasant with our patients. If she has one fault it is that she runs about 5 minutes late. However, her productivity and pleasantness more than make up for it. We've found her to be a wonderful colleague, and I trust you will too.

Some people write short letters of recommendation. Figure 11-3 is an example of a concise letter.

FIGURE 11-3

Short Recommendation Letter

Dear Dr. Rodriguez:

This is a letter of recommendation for Mary Smith, who is applying for your pharmacy technician position.

Mary has worked with me for 5 years. She recently went back to school to finish her pharmacy technician certification program. I was not surprised to learn that she did very well in the program, as she has done here for the past 5 years. Mary is energetic and diligent, and she works well with patients. I trust you will find her to be as admirable an employee as we have. We certainly will miss her.

Sincerely,

John Kim

Figure 11-4 (page 152) is an example of a letter of rec-ommendation for pharmacy school. Note how this letter ad-dresses the applicant's motivation, drive, time management, and personality in the context of the writer's work relationship with the applicant. This approach gives the reader a fuller understanding of the writer's perspective on the applicant. Such a letter is personal and more helpful than a standard-ized letter.

In some letters of recommendation, you may need to read between the lines. The words of a sophisticated writer can appear to be more positive than they actually are. Think about the implications of these two statements:

▌ I can't recommend this person highly enough.
▌ I can't recommend this person too highly.

The first statement implies that the prospective employee is so fantastic that the recommendation won't measure up to the employee's abilities. However, what if it means that the writer can't recommend this person highly enough *to be con-sidered for this position?* In the second statement, does it mean the person is highly qualified, or does it mean the person is average or even below par? Thus, it is important to read the entire letter to look for examples of behaviors or attributes to support one possible interpretation or the other.

Letters of recommendation and references are only part of the picture when you are hiring. Don't rely too heavily on them. Interview prospective employees long enough to form your own opinions. Weigh all the facts and then make a decision.

Training New Staff

The most important step for ensuring the success of new hires is to insist on adequate training. While many businesses prefer experience, it is not a substitute for intense training on your systems and operating procedures. A new hire should be given both written material and hands-on one-on-one experience with a veteran employee.

Written material with time to read through it and an op-portunity to ask questions is a valuable part of training. The very fact that someone took the time to write information

FIGURE 11-4

Letter of Recommendation for Pharmacy School

Re: Letter of recommendation for Michael Smith

Dear Admissions Committee:

It gives me great pleasure to introduce and recommend Michael Smith to your program. He possesses some outstanding traits that attest to his qualifications as a future pharmacist.

I met Michael when he came to my office looking for an opportunity to shadow a working pharmacist. This is not a normal program for our department. I told him that I would be happy to have him shadow me as long as he signed up for a program I'm involved in that is part volunteer and part mentorship. Michael lost no time in making this happen.

Michael has been working with me for the past 6 months. He is always prompt, dressed appropriately, and eager and willing to learn or help with whatever needs to be done. He is sensitive to the needs of others, including mine, and voluntarily assists in relieving my burden, which in turn frees up time for teaching him. However, Michael does not operate with a selfish outlook. During rounds (which is not usually an option for undergraduates), Michael has endeared himself to the team so much that they ask me where he is when he's not working with me. While eager to learn and experience things, he is not intrusive or inappropriate in other ways.

Michael's manners are impeccable without being excessive. He mixes well in all the pharmacy and medical circles I have taken him into, including patient training sessions. He is empathetic to the needs and experiences of others. His dedication to his studies is definitely present, but unlike other students, he can study *and* keep his work commitments. He's down to earth, modest, and yet visibly eager to get his hands wet in working as a pharmacist. His verbal communication skills are in the top 1%–5% of students. His written communication skills are also top-notch.

If you are looking for genuine people to help others with their medication needs, then Michael is the ideal candidate. Any school would be proud to have him as a student and as an alumnus.

Sincerely,

Cynthia Johnston

down signals that it is important. Moreover, having material in writing allows trainees to confirm information, absorb it at their own pace, and review it. If the same information is only transmitted verbally, trainees are likely to miss some key points. Of course, key areas of written material should be reviewed orally and with demonstration if applicable. This is particularly important with multistep tasks and functions for which you have a particular protocol.

Testing Competency

Once new employees have been given the policies and procedures portion of the training, it is appropriate to test them by requiring that they demonstrate the correct procedure instead of just reciting it. If technicians are reviewing your hospital policy on cassette fill, have them fill a section and check it for accuracy and completeness. If they are learning to transmit third-party claims, have them do so under supervision. If the skill needed is determining the quantity of medication to give for a prescription of a particular duration, have them perform the calculation. All these skills can be evaluated both in hypothetical test situations and in real situations, depending on your operation's need for documentation and the availability of testers or evaluators. However, actual demonstration when feasible provides a better indication of how well a person performs a given task.

Do not forget to assess verbal skills if they are necessary for the job function. If a new person is going to be taking refill requests off a message machine, then one way to determine competency is by having the new hire retrieve the refill requests and have a seasoned employee do the same thing. Then compare the two lists. Having the person answer a mock call from a nurse, doctor, or patient will determine whether the preferred image of your operation is actually being conveyed. Well-done coaching following a skills assessment can improve performance where training has fallen short.

How long should training last? The quick answer is that if you're usually impatient, figure it will take double the amount of time you think it should. If you tend to be forgiving, it should be no more than 3 to 6 months. Be assured that the person will not be following someone else during the entire apprenticeship. After the formal training of 2 to 4 weeks to

Periodic feedback is important— comments at an annual performance review should never be a surprise.

learn policies and procedures and the basic components of the job assignment in your arena, there will be a period of time during which the person should be able to perform most assignments unassisted but will need help should some unusual issues arise.

Periodic Assessment of Skills

Skill competency should be assessed regularly. The saying "Use it or lose it" certainly applies to pharmacy work. A certain set of minimum skills should be maintained by all personnel who might perform a particular job function. Yet, a technician who used to fill prescriptions but is now the key insurance adjudicator may no longer be up to par in dose calculations. So, look among the people you have and determine what types of competencies need to be available in case of emergency. Make sure the people who might be called on to use particular skills actually have them.

Competency assessment should be performed by someone who is familiar with the task and who regularly performs it. Providing a handout or review of the expectations before the evaluation is appropriate, especially in cases where some of the information may not have been used for some time. The opportunity to review the material before testing serves two purposes. First, it reminds the technician of the proper way a task is supposed to be done. Second, it educates someone who may have forgotten how or why a certain procedure is done. The opportunity to review makes the testing more fruitful. The purpose is to maintain a minimum skill level in order to protect patients, not to punish employees.

Feedback on Performance

It is a good idea to keep your employees aware of your opinion of their work. Some bosses are overly involved in day-to-day activities. This approach is known as micromanagement. These managers are so engrossed in the operation that they end up doing most of the work. A good supervisor has just enough participation in the day-to-day operation to understand its complexities, the challenges the staff faces, and the capabilities of each employee.

Periodic feedback is important—comments at an annual performance review should never be a surprise. The most effective feedback is given in a quiet, private setting where the supervisor and the employee can discuss issues. Short of the ability to sit down with every employee, a good practice is to praise openly and criticize privately.

To praise publicly, you must be genuine and selective. If you decide one day that everyone needs a morale boost and you therefore find something positive to say to each employee, you will only diminish the value of the compliments. Conversely, if you reserve praise for rare occasions, office morale will suffer. Find positive things to point out periodically so that people feel appreciated.

ACTIVITY

Here's an example of positive feedback from a supervisor: "John, I was very pleased with the way you handled Mrs. Jones. She can be very difficult. You sent her away smiling." Notice that the supervisor gave a compliment and also described the positive behavior.

Suppose the supervisor had said, "John, great job with Mrs. Jones. Thanks." Would the message communicated to John be any different? Think about how you give employees positive feedback. Phrase a work compliment in a way that reinforces the desired behavior.

Giving Negative Feedback

When it is necessary to give negative feedback, you should do so behind closed doors. Invite the employee into your office. In delivering bad news, such as the fact that you are not happy with the person's work, you might sandwich the facts between upbeat information to help focus the person and prevent a defeated attitude. For example: "Mary, I want you to know that I appreciate how well you organize the work area. It sure is a lot easier to find our supplies thanks to you. I am a little disappointed, however, in the speed with which you fill prescriptions. I know you are dedicated to the pharmacy, so I was wondering how you think this could improve?" Such an approach pumps up Mary at the outset, states the issue of concern, and invites Mary's input into the solution.

Formal Performance Reviews

A review is an opportunity to evaluate and document an employee's performance. It should not be a surprise to the employee. A fair review acknowledges the employee's accomplishments, praises outstanding behavior, and sets goals for future performance.

The supervisor's concerns should be known for the most part by both parties before a formal annual or semiannual review. Regular feedback reinforces expectations and provides the employee with an opportunity to improve in areas where there may be a deficit.

Some supervisors request that employees rate themselves first. If you elect to do this, spend some time evaluating the person beforehand so that you are prepared to discuss discrepancies. Ask the employee to make a list of accomplishments over the year, since you may not remember or be aware of everything. In addition, be open enough to consider the employee's opinion, which may differ from your own, and strong enough to refute an inflated self-evaluation with facts. Give suggestions for growth and areas for the employee to work on for the coming year.

Delivering Unpleasant News

Unwelcome news, particularly news related to discipline or firing, should be delivered in a confidential setting. The employee receiving it may become emotional and argumentative. Many institutions have a policy requiring two managers to deliver this kind of news. Other times, you may be communicating negative news solo.

Once the decision has been made to discipline or fire someone, it is best given succinctly and with supporting data. For instance, if someone is constantly late, it is wise to show the employee actual time-clock data that support this statement. Figure 11-5 provides an example of a warning letter.

FIGURE 11-5

Warning Letter

Dear Ms. Sutherland:

This is a letter of warning regarding your attendance. You have failed to report to work within the designated time period on multiple occasions. On June 12, you clocked in at 9:10 am for a 9 o'clock shift. On June 14, you clocked in at 9:23 am, and on June 23, you arrived at 9:18 am.

It is the departmental policy that you arrive no later than 5 minutes after 9:00 am. Failure to do so will result in additional action up to and including termination.

You are a valuable member of our team. We rely on your work to ensure that our patients get the best care. I trust that you will make arrangements to correct this situation.

Sincerely,

Janet Roberts

Assignment Changes and Skill Development

One of the responsibilities of a supervisor is determining what skills are needed and who is most capable in a particular role. It is the supervisor's job to help employees do their best and achieve their ultimate jobs.

You should be aware that just because you want to be a boss doesn't mean that every employee wants to be one. Some want a different challenge or environment. Your job as the boss is to sort this out and help employees achieve their particular goals. First, though, you have to help employees be the best assistants for you. The first step is to get them the necessary training. Sometimes it means giving people the opportunity to grow with a new challenge.

Identifying why a person is receiving training goes a long way toward reducing rumors. Open and honest communication is important. Let's look at some ways to approach the news that a technician will be getting additional training.

Situation 1

Everyone from the satellite pharmacies is going to be cross-trained in the sterile-products department to allow for greater flexibility in staffing. In this case, the announcement that the cross-training will occur can be made in a staff meeting with everyone present. A schedule can be created. The duration of training for each individual and the amount of time the whole process is estimated to take should be shared as well.

One of the pitfalls of giving a time frame and a schedule is that often in health care, things come up and the project never gets completed. But without a time frame, employees become disenchanted and rumors start.

Situation 2

There will be some job reassignments in the pharmacy. At the moment, you are not at liberty to share these with the staff. One key position will change, and it is necessary to train someone to assume that role. You pick the second most productive employee in the department to take on this new role because it requires a lot of detail work. This person is good at detail, and you don't want to lose your best producer to this less demanding role. Your choice for the position will work well without a lot of supervision.

The best way to break this news is to arrange a meeting to inform the person who will receive the training. You might say, "You're doing a good job for us in the inpatient department. We need to train another person in the narcotics vault. Because you have such good attention to detail, you would be very good in this position. I thought you might be interested in this new challenge."

You don't owe an explanation to the people not chosen for the role. But if there is a way to explain your decision and convey your confidence in them as well, doing so can go a long way toward maintaining morale and commitment. For instance, you might discuss with your top performer or a veteran employee that you are making some changes. You could note that you want to keep the person's good skills to make sure the operation keeps running efficiently. If there are going to be more opportunities in the future, you might mention this, but don't make the mistake of promising a role that might never materialize. It's also not a good idea to make excuses to make someone feel better. If the people not getting the new position are interested in expanding their roles, you might take the opportunity to encourage their growth and point them in a direction of skill building that would be useful to your organization.

If you are cross-training someone for a role where the current person in the role might feel threatened by someone else being able to perform the task, you might tell both that certain tasks are essential and you want to make sure that you can cover the assignments if the current person is out. Often, the best person to train someone is the person in the role. By including the current employee in the process, you show a certain amount of trust in that person's competence. Of course, if the current person isn't performing well and the intent is to replace him or her, you need to weigh whether you or the current person should be the trainer. You don't want to have bad habits passed on.

Human Resources Department

Most organizations have human resources (HR) departments that are particularly helpful to management. HR employees are specially trained in areas of staff management and training. Larger companies provide leadership and managerial workshops taught by HR staff. The HR department may also be available to give coaching or hints for conducting interviews, handling staff issues, writing schedules, conducting meetings, and disciplining employees.

The personnel in human resources can also help guide you in legal matters. Often, certain procedures must be followed in sensitive cases, such as firing or counseling a staff member when behavior is unacceptable. Additionally, in many shops, union contracts dictate how these issues are to be handled. Contracts may have policies about written warnings, such as what language they must contain. Generally, written warnings are given to employees after verbal counseling has failed to produce results. For instance, let's say an employee is consistently late. After bringing this to the employee's attention verbally, the employee still fails to arrive as scheduled over 50% of the time. At this point, it becomes necessary to

Recognition of a job well done goes far toward improving trust between the manager and employees.

document that you have had a conversation about timeliness with the employee. Within this documentation, you need to succinctly spell out what is expected. Some HR departments have specific rules on how to write these letters and may provide templates for you.

Management Styles

There are different types of bosses. Adjusting your management style to complement the personalities of your employees helps create a more favorable work environment. Self-discovery will help you temper your personality to get the most from your employees with their cooperation rather than just their desire to keep their jobs.

Some bosses feel they need control, so they prefer to dictate exactly how every operation will be performed. They work in predictable environments that function well until something unplanned occurs, such as too many people calling in sick. They tend to micromanage, eliminating room for their employees to think for themselves and solve problems.

Other bosses are conceptual. Sometimes this is a good thing and sometimes not. They give few or no specifics on the method to accomplish work tasks or what a project is to look like in the end. People who have this style need to be aware that without good communication, a finished product may look quite different from what they conceived, even though the function is the same. On the positive side, such a management style often allows employees to explore new ways to present things. It provides managers with an opportunity to expand their realm of possibilities. Such freedom to create, however, can also lead to disappointment for a manager with distinct ideas about how things should be done.

Each manager has a style. Self-awareness is an important asset because it allows you to adjust how you relate to individuals enough to be successful without compromising who you are.

Communication and feedback are important. If there are specifications for a project, they need to be communicated to the people carrying out the assignment before it is completed. Waiting until the final product is presented to express dissatisfaction or desired changes may lead to a waste of resources, time, and spirit, as well as to hard feelings. Recognition of a job well done goes far toward improving trust between the manager and employees.

Managing Productive Staff

The following example illustrates how a manager's expectations can hinder productivity.

A conceptual boss gave a pharmacist who was a model employee an assignment that involved setting up a new mail-order home-care operation. The boss provided little direction. The outcome was an efficient operation in a production area, with a predictable and predetermined amount of work each day. On rare occasions, last-minute orders occurred.

The model employee was able to complete all tasks early in the morning with the designated staff. Because of the physical remoteness of the operation, it was not feasible for the staff of this part of the operation to help out in one of the other pharmacies. As a result, the staff was left to wait for any last-minute orders. Everything that needed to get done, including advance preparations, was always finished without overtime. The pharmacist read pharmacy texts in most of the spare time, but on occasion he read the newspaper or a magazine during downtime.

Eventually the boss discovered what was happening. Instead of giving the area additional assignments, the model employee was relocated to a busier area. Another pharmacist was brought in to head the operation. Because she was able to make the same amount of work last the whole day, the boss was much happier with her performance.

Penalizing efficiency does not improve the performance of an operation. It demoralizes good employees and eventually costs the operation by requiring extra personnel. As a manager, it is your job to be explicit and divide the work among your staff. If the area lacks work, the problem is not with the staff members.

In the case mentioned above, the manager's actions resulted in the assigned work taking all day to complete. When volume increased, so did the need for staff and consequently the cost to run the operation. The lesson: don't be so rigid that the staff works against you to reduce their productivity.

Maintaining a Pleasant Work Environment

Many bosses bring in goodies periodically to add cheer to the workplace. Others celebrate birthdays or other holidays to boost morale. Bagels in the morning or scones at coffee provide a treat for employees and work well when the boss is also perceived as caring and kind. When the boss is not respected, they only provide a free meal and a subject of mockery.

Bringing in goodies such as donuts on a scheduled day every week promotes a positive expectation. Expectations, though, can become "rights," and not providing them can cause disappointment. But bringing in unexpected treats because the team has been working hard, just finished a tough week, or implemented a new system becomes a reward and is usually perceived as part of a work environment where the boss appreciates the efforts of subordinates.

Everyone likes cake, and birthdays are a great way to honor someone and provide a snack for employees. All birthdays, however, should be celebrated in a similar manner. Otherwise, these occasions can divide the staff and cause resentments. People who get "better" birthdays are perceived as favored, and others with less special celebrations may feel slighted.

How would it look if one month the boss took a staff member out to lunch alone on his birthday but the next month brought in a cake for another staff member? It may be that in the first instance, the boss simply forgot to order a cake, and buying lunch seemed like a reasonable alternative. However, the second person may think that lunch is a special 90-minute celebration and the cake is only a routine obligation. Consistency avoids unnecessary grievances and the resentment they breed.

Consistency also eliminates seasonal differences over which you have no control. Birthdays occurring in holiday-free August might provide a welcome opportunity to celebrate, but December birthdays might be lost among the holiday parties. By the time mid-August rolls around, people who took early summer vacations or those who aren't going to take one are eager for any occasion to celebrate. Come December, people might be tired of parties. Fellow employees working to clean things up for the new year might not miss the additional cake, but the guest of honor would. For these reasons, it's a good idea to find a way to celebrate birthdays consistently. Some work groups find having a monthly celebration more feasible than individual parties. Other groups find that rotating the host is a good way to share the burden and ensure participation. Let your staff members determine the best way for them to celebrate.

All the cake in the world does not compensate for a disrespectful and unpleasant work environment. A boss who taunts employees or who has unrealistic expectations of what can be accomplished in a period of time will not create happy employees simply by buying food. A boss who chats on the phone all day while the rest of the staff is working to fill orders and deliver medications to the nursing stations will not win friends by organizing social events. Social events enhance an already good work environment. They do not make up for otherwise bad working conditions.

A seasoned manager can help reduce conflicts and settle small disagreements before they become insurmountable.

ACTIVITY

Identify ways that you can show your appreciation to your staff. Does it always need to involve food or money?

Internal Conflict Prevention and Management

In any situation where people are close to one another for extended periods of time, conflicts are going to develop. This is true of family relationships and friendships. Everyone has experienced interpersonal conflicts, such as sibling rivalry, disagreements between parents, and neighborhood spats. When issues evoke feelings such as jealousy, resentment, or disappointment, there is apt to be conflict.

A seasoned manager can help reduce conflicts and settle small disagreements before they become insurmountable. One way to keep the peace is to be aware of what is happening in your area of responsibility. Stay alert for hints of problems. Keeping your door open to hear employees' issues and welcoming pop-in conversations are great ways to learn about potential problems. Of course, a good manager can ferret out a real problem from a venting session. Nonetheless, being made aware of an issue early on allows you to plan a resolution before it develops into a bigger problem.

Sometimes a suggestion box can help identify areas of concern that employees are unwilling to talk about with you. At times, it may be preferable to confront a situation directly by asking those affected to participate in a resolution session.

Let's look at a scenario involving two employees at the same organization. One employee always comes to work in a jovial mood. While signing in, she inquires about everyone's weekend or discusses the previous night's television shows. Afterward, she flits around the pharmacy, getting coffee and checking the bulletin board. The second employee feels that his colleague is wasting time. He starts working immediately. He usually arrives a little early and is engaged in the day's work at starting time.

Resentment builds in the second employee. Eventually, he starts to complain. From your perspective, both do an adequate job, although the output of the complainer might be slightly greater than that of the jovial employee. At the end of the day, the first employee leaves on time. The other employee waits to make sure that everything is in order for the next shift. After some time, the complainer makes it clear that he does not enjoy working with the jovial employee.

You pull the two into your office to discuss the matter. In such situations, it may be best to be a mediator, allowing the two employees to work out a resolution and not dictating one yourself. Following are two examples of how the conversation might go.

Example 1

Supervisor (you): There seems to be some ill feelings developing between you two. Can you help me understand what is going on?

Employee 2 (complainer): She doesn't do her fair share of work. She comes in and dilly-dallies for half an hour while the rest of us are working. I don't need Susie Sunshine first thing in the morning.

Supervisor: It seems to me that you need some quiet time in the morning. [Note: The supervisor did not argue the point about productivity. Evaluating work output is the supervisor's job.]

Employee 2: Yes I do. It's distracting to have someone bounce into work when we have all these orders to do.

Supervisor: It sounds like you would be happier if she would arrive at work more quietly and wait until later in the morning to talk with you.

Employee 2: Well at least I'd know she was helping. The way it is now, she acts like this is some kind of party.

Supervisor (to employee 1): Do you think you could be a little less talkative first thing in the morning? We all have a lot of work to get done. Having some of it finished before we start socializing will probably relieve some of the pressure he is feeling.

Employee 1: I can try.

Supervisor (to employee 2): Will that work for you?

Employee 2: I think so.

Supervisor (to employee 2): Maybe you could cut her some slack by saying hello.

In this case, you have taken control of the conversation. Instead of allowing the two employees to argue with each other, you have preempted a conversation about work quality and other habits and led the conversation to the immediate issue. Let's see how this conversation could get out of hand.

Example 2
Supervisor (you): There seems to be some ill feeling developing between you two. Can you help me understand what is going on?

Employee 2 (complainer): She doesn't do her fair share of work. She comes in and dilly-dallies for half an hour while the rest of us are working. I don't need Susie Sunshine first thing in the morning.

Employee 1: At least I don't come in as Old Sourpuss. You don't even say hello.

Employee 2: I wasn't hired as a cheerleader. We have patients to take care of, but you just think it's one big party.

In this example, the two employees are fighting with each other. This type of discussion goes nowhere. By the time you get involved, your first objective will be changing the subject, not furthering the resolution as in example 1.

Personnel issues are challenging and require skill to resolve. Building your communication skills will help you feel comfortable in dealing with them. Often, successful managers rehearse various scenarios so that the communication is second nature when they are presented with a challenge.

Summary

Staff management involves hiring, scheduling, and creating a pleasant work environment with reasonable policies and procedures. In addition, training, counseling, and evaluating performance are key components of staff management. Hiring requires careful review of a potential employee's written presentation (the application and résumé) and personal attributes (the interview and references). Usable references may be difficult to obtain—and to provide—because many companies have restrictive policies on what may be said.

Staff management involves an ongoing commitment to ensuring employees' skill competency. To do this, initial training and periodic evaluation of competency are necessary. Evaluation can be done by demonstration—that is, watching while someone performs a task. It can also be done by written or verbal examination when the focus is on retained knowledge.

Giving periodic feedback is important so that employees do not have to guess about what you expect and will not be surprised during annual performance evaluations. Good work should be recognized as often as possible. When there are areas requiring improvement, the manager should discuss them with the employee privately and empathetically and provide coaching. A fair review acknowledges an employee's accomplishments, praises outstanding behavior, and sets goals for future performance.

Social events create a better atmosphere in an already good atmosphere. Managers need to maintain a positive environment and resolve conflicts immediately so that resentments don't fester. In short, managers are responsible for ensuring that there is an adequate number of competent staff members and that they work in the most positive environment possible.

For More Information

Brown KR. Development of a work-force retention program. *Am J Health Syst Pharm.* 2008;65(1):20–1.

Desselle SP, Vaughan M, Faria T. Creating a performance appraisal template for pharmacy technicians using the method of equal-appearing intervals. *J Am Pharm Assoc.* 2002;42(5):768–79.

Mahoney CD, Gallina JN, Jeffrey LP. A comprehensive program to increase job satisfaction among pharmacy technicians. *Hosp Pharm.* 1982;17(10):547–50.

Pershing JA. *Handbook of Human Performance Technology.* 3rd ed. San Francisco: Pfeiffer; 2006.

CHAPTER | 12

Team Building, Coaching, and Mentoring

Rarely can someone do all tasks alone and well. In most operations, we rely on one another to share the work. We hope that the people we share work with are pleasant and make the work environment enjoyable. We also hope that we can trust others to help us out when we are overburdened. This is called teamwork.

Teamwork doesn't happen automatically. Let's look at some of the language of professional sports and the team approach. In baseball, one statistic is RBI, or runs batted in. Notice that it isn't "runs made." By nature, the term "runs batted in" credits one team member with contributing to the successful outcome of other team members' hits to contribute to the team's total score. In basketball and ice hockey, the concept is called "assists." The men and women who play these team sports practice together. They are taught to understand the importance of the other players and learn to trust one another.

Likewise, in a business setting such as a pharmacy, teamwork requires respect and trust, as well as training and practice. Cross-training, or learning one another's specific job functions, allows each person to work in the different roles in a pharmacy. When someone is overwhelmed, another can chip in.

Teamwork in pharmacies also involves respect for individual abilities. Sometimes it isn't chipping in that is necessary but delegating responsibilities to the most appropriate person on the basis of skill or availability. For instance, one person might be chosen to represent the pharmacy at a particular meeting. The reason might be the shift the person is working, a skill the person has, or the fact that the person is not as essential to the operation at that time as others are. Whatever the reason, the rest of the staff may have to cover work normally done by that person.

Teamwork requires respect and trust, as well as training and practice.

Building a team helps improve morale and move the operation forward. But many things can get in the way of a team attitude. They include the following:

▌ Petty jealousy
▌ Lack of motivation of one member of the group
▌ Sabotage—intentional actions to interfere with success
▌ Discontent in the group
▌ Disrespect for one another
▌ Poor work habits
▌ Lack of interest
▌ Lack of caring
▌ Lack of knowledge of each other

It's difficult to bring people into a room and dictate that they will all work well together. There are some methods that can help break down barriers to team building.

First, colleagues should get to know one another. A way to facilitate this is to break people into groups and have them introduce themselves. Then, have a person from each group introduce the group members to the gathering as a whole. Usually this activity works best if there is a theme to the introductions, such as hobbies, where you went to school, what kind of jobs you have had, or how long you have been working for the company.

Second, people have to be invested in the process for it to work. In a work environment, the need for a job is one way that everyone is invested, but this can fizzle if the team falters. A sense of pride in the work done or the accomplishment of the group can be nurtured and lead to team success. Recognition of individual contributions to the team shows that each person is valued. Celebration of achievements helps show appreciation and confirm the importance of the team's work.

While it's important to show appreciation for individual work, favoritism leads to discontent and mistrust. You don't want to reward someone just because it's his or her turn, but if you focus your appreciation on only a few people, only the favorites and the self-motivated will contribute their all. The rest will just get by.

Meetings

Meetings are great ways to bring people and their ideas together. It is important that they occur frequently enough to keep everyone informed of important developments, but news is not the only reason to have a meeting. Soliciting staff ideas for solutions to problems or for new projects is a way to generate the feeling that everyone is an important and contributing part of the team.

Before calling a meeting, the chairperson should be clear about the objective. The agenda should include items that will accomplish this. If possible, an agenda should be set with the input of the attendees. Some managers like to set the first part of the agenda and also leave time for an open-discussion section during which others can bring their concerns to the table. An efficient way to run a meeting is for the agenda to include estimated time and desired outcomes. Figure 12-1 is an example of an agenda that incorporates these items.

FIGURE 12-1

Example of an Agenda

Agenda
Staff Meeting: April 10, 2009

Topic	Speaker	Outcome	Time
Computer update	Susie	Informational	10 min
New hours	Susie	Decision	15 min
Vacation schedule	All	Decisions	20 min
Open discussion	All	Discuss other topics	10 min

Once the agenda is set and the participants have been notified of the time and place, it's time to think about how you want to approach the meeting. If you truly want discussion, then all the participants have to be made to feel as though their input is important. Even a shy person has something to say, and a good moderator can bring it out. When you are just making announcements, make it clear ahead of time that discussion is not needed. Understand that cutting off discussion may cause discontent and "underground" conversations.

Leading a meeting requires more than just getting through the agenda items. It is important to keep everyone engaged, invite participation, and prevent the meeting from getting sidetracked. There are many good books with hints on running effective meetings.

Meetings can get sidetracked in many ways. For example, sometimes enthusiastic staff members veer off topic during a discussion, or they bring up items they feel are important before the set agenda is completed. You want to avoid a runaway meeting, but controlling such digressions is tricky. Stopping conversation too quickly may stifle future openness. But allowing a discussion not pertaining to the agenda topics may prevent the group from completing its business. If consensus cannot be reached in a timely manner, you may have to end the discussion in order to get through the planned agenda. Offering to discuss the topic later in the meeting or to put it on a future agenda is a good strategy. Then you must do that.

For topics where you want consensus, the group may have a variation on your idea. Sometimes a manager doesn't understand this, and the staff becomes disenchanted.

A number of years ago, a manager wanted support for remodeling the pharmacy, so she called a meeting. The invitation read, "Help plan the new pharmacy. All interested parties welcome." At the meeting, it became apparent that the discussion would go on until the participants agreed with what the manager wanted to do. Many of the staff decided not to join the planning committee. The moral of the story: if you solicit opinions, be open to considering them.

When you run a meeting, try to stay within the allotted time. Be respectful of attendees' time. If it is necessary to run over, ask permission to do so and acknowledge that you understand if some cannot stay. Meetings that repeatedly run over should be scheduled for a longer time or run with tighter control by staying on topic.

It is a good idea to summarize what was discussed at the meeting before adjourning. In this way, all the decisions are fresh in everyone's mind, and any differences in understanding can be resolved.

Finally, get the minutes typed up and distributed to everyone who was invited as soon as possible after the meeting. The minutes remind participants of the meeting's key information, decisions, and action items, and they also help inform those who could not attend.

Coaching and Mentoring

What is coaching and mentoring? Let's first talk about adult learning styles.

Adults learn in many different ways. Some people are conceptual, learning best by reading a theory and applying it. Others are literal. They need specific, step-by-step instructions. Other adults are visual learners. They need a picture—for example, a graph or table—of the subject matter. Still others learn best through demonstration. Finally, some people prefer to figure things out for themselves. These are the ones whom you mentor. Point them in the direction you want them to go, and let them learn on their own.

In mentoring, you help subordinates recognize opportunities and develop to their fullest potential. Some managers fear that they might be replaced if a subordinate becomes too good. Actually, that should be your goal—you also should be moving upward in your organization or toward new and different challenges.

A mentor needs a good sense of the mentee's goals. This understanding is achieved through discussion. The mentor may also propose options that the mentee has not considered. Once the interests are established, the mentor identifies opportunities to expand the mentee's horizons in those areas. Examples include pointing out relevant seminars and conferences, providing opportunities to shadow people involved in the area of interest, and discussing articles about topics of interest. A mentor can also help the mentee examine his or her experiences and learn from them.

Mentoring develops a person for career advancement. Mentors encourage, coach, evaluate, listen, and question. They provide challenges that help mentees acquire new skills. They coax mentees to take advantage of opportunities. They help mentees overcome doubts. And mentors often find leads for their mentees' next positions.

In coaching, you help employees be the best they are capable of being. One technique is to lead people to discover on their own what you want them to learn. Of course, you will need to lead some employees a little more directly to the

Mentors encourage, coach, evaluate, listen, and question.

point of discovery, but the best ones will be quite capable of finding answers independently.

Sometimes coaching is done to help employees perform assigned tasks with greater success. Other times, it is to teach them new skills to enhance their job satisfaction, expand their responsibilities, or change their assignments. Let's look at a few ways you can achieve successful coaching sessions.

To begin, determine the goal of the session. What is it that you want the employee to learn, or what skill would you like to develop? Why is it that the skill needs improvement?

Coaching is a way of giving feedback, but it also has a plan of action. You should be warm and open so that the employee is receptive, not defensive. In corrective coaching, think through the issue. You should be able to describe how the employee's performance is unsatisfactory or what skill you want the employee to develop. Let's consider two examples:

1. A work performance problem: "John, I'd like to discuss your cassette filling. There have been quite a few errors lately. I'm concerned about your accuracy level. How can I help you improve it?"

2. Career development: "John, you've been working here for nine years. You've always done a good job for us with cassette fill. I'd like you to take on more responsibility in the area of ordering. How might we make that happen?"

In both cases, you should let the employee respond so that you are sure he or she understands why you are raising the issue and what you expect. Once you get the feedback, work out specific activities and a timetable to achieve the goals and measure progress. Involving the employee in developing the goals with you rather than dictating them builds a working relationship and fosters buy-in. It also helps the employee develop a learning plan, a skill that can be applied in future situations. If, before the review time, you observe that the goals are not being met, you should give feedback to get the employee on track.

One way to be successful in coaching is by asking questions that help the employee recognize the issue and contribute ideas to fix it. You are coaching the employee into identifying the changes that need to be made and often the way to make them. You become the cheerleader, guide, and facilitator of the change.

Generating Respect Upward

The boss gets respect initially because he or she is the boss. By showing favoritism, making poor decisions, failing to help the team when things get tough, or acting particularly moody, the boss loses the team's respect. With too many such errors, the boss risks losing control of the team. Some people will still do their jobs, but the camaraderie of the group will vanish.

Bosses need to be accessible while still being able to get their own work done. An open-door policy invites honest discussion with an emphasis on performance improvement. A helping hand to the team shows that the boss respects the work the employees are doing—and in turn generates respect for the boss.

Helping out does not mean doing the work for the team. In one operation, for example, a particular manager was well liked. Instead of allowing the employees to do their jobs and coaching those who underperformed, the manager filled remaining orders and cleaned up loose ends daily. When the manager left, the team remained dysfunctional, and output suffered. A good boss helps out but doesn't take on the tasks. A good boss coaches to achieve required outcomes.

ACTIVITY

Suppose that someone from another department complains. From what the supervisor hears, the complaint seems valid.

How might each of the following responses sound to the person complaining? How might they sound to a member of the supervisor's team? How might they sound to the person who is the target of the complaint?

- "I'll talk to my employee and straighten this out."
- "I'll have a word with my employee. Ugh."
- "Let me talk to my employee and find out what happened."
- "It seems to me you are upset about [the action]. How would we do things differently to please you next time?"

A leader inspires others to develop the tasks needed to attain the goals.

Respect is also earned by actions. It can be earned when the boss sticks up for employees when they are right, supports the operation when necessary, and obtains needed resources, such as money, help, or supplies.

Leadership versus Management

Many scholarly articles discuss the difference between management and leadership. Some people use the two terms interchangeably, assuming that a person in a management position must also be a leader. There are implied differences between the two. *Fortune Magazine* described the differences this way: "The manager administers, the leader innovates. The manager maintains, the leader develops. The manager relies on systems, the leader relies on people. The manager counts on controls, the leader counts on trust. The manager does things right, the leader does the right thing."[1]

The differences between a manager and a leader can be described in other ways as well. A manager focuses on achieving a defined set of goals with the available people and supplies. A leader has a vision and defines the goals. A manager assigns the people he is given to the tasks at hand. A leader inspires others to develop the tasks needed to attain the goals. A manager evaluates success on the basis of completing tasks and complying with policy. A leader measures success on the basis of meeting aspiration with attainment, learning from mistakes, and inspiring to achieve, grow, and innovate.

This is not to suggest that a leader is a dreamer and a manager is a doer. To the contrary, both work toward goals. The power of leadership is that through innovation comes development and growth. Leaders create an environment that is exciting and vibrant. They look for ways to guide and build to new levels.

What kind of a boss do you want to be?

Summary

Being a boss is more than filling out paperwork, assigning tasks, and accounting for employees. One of the most rewarding aspects of management is motivating and helping team members to pursue their goals. The boss first needs to create an environment that stimulates productivity and growth. This is usually done by building a team attitude among co-workers. Helping employees fulfill their potential and attain their goals may require inspiring them through mentoring, or it may require coaching them to improve their skills and work habits. A good manager develops his or her mentoring and coaching skills to be able to guide the staff toward success.

Reference

1. Brown HJ Jr. *A Father's Book of Wisdom*. Nashville, Tenn: Rutledge Hill Press; 1988:78.

For More Information

Bross RA, Ness JE, Rudisill R. Benefits of forming pharmacy technician teams. *Am J Health Syst Pharm.* 2004;61(13):1389–91.

Lee MP, Ray MD. Planning for pharmaceutical care. *Am J Hosp Pharm.* 1993;50(6):1153–8.

Lundin SC, Paul H, Christensen J. *Fish! A Remarkable Way to Boost Morale and Improve Results.* New York: Hyperion; 2000.

Shane RR. Pharmacy without walls. *Am J Health Syst Pharm.* 1996;53(4):418–25.

Wageman R, Nunes D, Burruss J, et al. *Senior Leadership Teams: What It Takes to Make Them Great.* Boston: Harvard Business School Press; 2008.

White SJ. Managing yourself so others want to work with you. *Am J Health Syst Pharm.* 2008;65(10):922–5.

Wollenburg K. Managing up, over, and across. *Am J Health Syst Pharm.* 2001;58 suppl 1:S10-3.

CHAPTER | 13

Selected Issues Affecting Pharmacy Practice

Health care is an ever-changing field. Over the course of a career, issues will arise that change practice models, the ways we treat diseases, the kind of health care a person can access and the extent of treatments, and payment structures. Over the past 50 years, for example, we have witnessed an enormous expansion of the types of drugs available to treat particular diseases. Hypertension could be treated with a few diuretics, one beta blocker, an alkaloid, and a handful of vasodilators in the early 1970s. Today, it can also be treated with calcium channel blockers, angiotensin-converting enzyme inhibitors (ACEs), and angiotensin receptor blockers (ARBs). Kidney failure was a death sentence in the middle of the last century, but hemodialysis and transplants have allowed many patients to live a decade or more after their initial diagnosis. Doctors, nurses, and pharmacists were the health care practitioners until the 1980s, when fields such as nurse practitioner, physician's assistant, and pharmacy technician emerged. Payment for services used to be fee based. Now, health care "memberships" in the form of prepaid HMOs is developing as the predominant financial model.

As you work in a health care field, it is important to be informed about various trends and ideas as they emerge. Reading articles and attending seminars where such issues are discussed and developed help prepare you for the inevitable changes. This chapter briefly discusses some current hot topics in the pharmacy field.

Tech-Check-Tech

As pharmacists take on more direct patient-care responsibilities, the profession of pharmacy has begun looking for ways to increase efficiency. Expanding the role of technicians is one new approach. Previously, technicians were authorized to perform certain routine functions in pharmacies under the direct supervision of pharmacists. Before any order or prescription filled by a technician could leave the pharmacy in any practice setting, it was checked by a pharmacist for accuracy. This, of course, required a pharmacist to be physically available where the technician was working—that is, in the pharmacy. A pharmacist bound to the pharmacy inhibits the communication and camaraderie necessary to develop interdisciplinary relationships that best serve patients.

To foster interdisciplinary relationships between pharmacists and other providers, pharmacists are exploring ways to free up their time. Of course, they realize that even the most ingenious pharmaceutical-care plan is worthless if the medication never reaches the patient. One way to achieve a balance is to give technicians more responsibility but still realize that only pharmacists have the training required to evaluate the risk versus the benefit of any particular order or prescription. Since many facilities use computerized physician order entry, or CPOE, verifying orders can be done remotely as long as a computer is available. With this in mind, some states have approved the use of technicians to check the preparation of orders, such as routine cassette filling done by other technicians. This system is called tech-check-tech.

Tech-check-tech accuracy was validated in a two-year trial.[1] In the trial, the technicians reviewing the cassette filling of other technicians were at least as accurate as pharmacists doing the same task. During the same time period, pharmacists in the test institutions were able to devote over an hour more a day to direct patient care. More institutions and states will likely implement such programs.

Medication Therapy Management

Medication therapy management (MTM) has been a goal of pharmaceutical services for decades. MTM is based on evidence that the cause of a large percentage of hospitalizations is multiple medications, or "poly-pharmacy." With the overhaul of Medicare, third-party payer compensation for MTM became a reality for pharmacists in 2006.

MTM is a required benefit of patients funded by Medicare. Officials decided that close monitoring of the medications that seniors and other Medicare recipients take would reduce the number of adverse incidents associated with medications in these populations. The success of this program no doubt will open the way for additional mandates for patients sponsored by other third parties.

What does this mean for technicians and pharmacists? For pharmacists, it means increased use of their clinical skills. As with any new program, although the data support the concept, it is important for pharmacists to show during the implementation period that they can deliver high-quality services. To ensure success, pharmacists need to redefine their roles and perhaps delegate more. For technicians, it means additional responsibilities to free up pharmacists' time for MTM consultations.

Change brings new challenges. Rising to the occasion can bring new career opportunities.

Technicians should be aware of who is entitled to these services and how to bill for them. Pharmacies may need to establish specific consultation hours. Some pharmacies may implement the program by appointment only, while others may deliver the services on a first-come, first-served basis. Either way, it will probably be technicians' responsibility to monitor use, ensure patient flow, and maintain order in providing these services.

As the program unfolds, additional services may be implemented or documentation requirements may be mandated. Staying on top of changes and being aware of how to document for billing will be roles for technicians. Technicians may also be given additional prescription preparation or refill responsibilities. It's important to understand that change brings new challenges. Rising to the occasion can bring new career opportunities.

Reimbursement

Relatively few workers are independently wealthy. For everyone else, jobs are necessary. For any business to survive, receipts—the money taken in—must cover expenses, including salaries and rent.

Reimbursement is a main topic of discussion at many pharmacy society meetings. The discussion focuses on two issues: adequate reimbursement for tangible services (that is, medications) being provided, including salary costs to prepare them, and reimbursement for professional services rendered, such as medication therapy management, pharmaceutical care, and consultations.

Today, most patients have a third-party payer, otherwise known as insurance, that pays part or all of their medical expenses. Those with public payers such as Medicaid have complete coverage. Those with private carriers pay part or all of a premium, as well as co-payments for covered services they receive.

Collecting reimbursement from the insurance company used to be the responsibility of the patient. The provider of services received payment in full from the patient and gave the patient a receipt. It was the patient's responsibility to submit the claim for reimbursement.

Now, claims are handled online, and most insurance companies have made deals with providers that reimburse at minimal levels. The so-called margin of profit barely covers the cost of keeping a store open, much less the salary of the pharmacist and technicians. Many of the contracts were initiated with chain-store pharmacies, which use the prescription business as a loss leader to bring people into the store. For independents, the pharmacy business is the key reason to bring people into the store. Unfortunately, many of these independent operations have been forced to close because managed-care contract reimbursement provisions are insufficient to cover basic costs.

Nonetheless, even for chain stores, hospital clinic pharmacies, and inpatient pharmacies, reimbursement for prescriptions and for medications used in hospitals has become an issue. Hospitals are often reimbursed according to diagnosis-related group (DRG) rates—that is, the diagnosis drives the rate of reimbursement, regardless of the treatment cost, length of stay (LOS), or a patient's complications, such as developing a nosocomial infection. With more and more expensive medications included in various standards of treatment, the DRG reimbursement is often inadequate.

Flaws with online adjudication systems also affect reimbursement for medications. Once approval is received online, the claim is supposed to be paid, but that does not always happen in practice. Pharmacies have reported getting corrections and inquiries after the fact. Answering these inquires or validating necessity is time-consuming and often not fruitful.

The second reimbursement issue is the recognition of professional pharmacist services. Historically, patients went to pharmacists for advice. Pharmacist-proprietors gave advice freely, in part to build relationships with patients and in part because the pricing of prescriptions was sufficient to compensate them comfortably. But the practice of pharmacy has changed.

Currently, pharmacists offer services that are not directly associated with products. MTM is one such service. Pharmacists monitor patient treatments, such as anticoagulation medications, asthma therapy, and antihypertensive therapy. In collaborative relationships with doctors, these pharmacists often write prescriptions and are independently responsible for the success of treatments. In some manner, they need to be compensated either directly or through the practice.

National societies and professional organizations are working with public and private payers to recognize the importance of these services and reimburse for them. The American Pharmacists Association (APhA) and the American Society of Health-System Pharmacists (ASHP) were instrumental in lobbying successfully for the recognition of pharmacists as providers of MTM through Medicare Part D services. A number of pharmacists have also successfully marketed services to self-paying patients who understand the benefit of pharmaceutical care in maximizing the outcome they can get from medications for controlling chronic diseases.

Technician Education and Certification
Historical Perspective
As independent pharmacy practice gave way to chain-store operations, the volume output demands made on pharmacists in larger facilities impaired their ability to act in the consultant role. During the same period, drug development exploded, increasing demand for the specialized medication knowledge that pharmacists possess. Even in hospital settings, providing pharmaceutical expertise was challenging when the pharmacy and staff were relegated to the basement.

Pharmacists began organizing to seek a larger role in therapeutic decisions and a return to counseling and patient interaction. But delivering pharmaceutical care and at the same time meeting a greatly increased level of tangible productivity were impossible without support help. Thus, trained people who could ably assist pharmacists were in demand.

The evolution of the technician's role followed the evolu-

Recognition that well-trained technicians could cover some of the straightforward roles previously held by pharmacists opened the door to pharmacy technology as a career.

tion of the pharmacist's role. As the need for the expertise of pharmacists expanded, health care delivery costs, including drug acquisition, salaries and benefits, and rent, rose. Creative solutions for getting the work done were needed. Recognition that well-trained technicians could cover some of the straightforward roles previously held by pharmacists opened the door to pharmacy technology as a career.

Originally, assistants working in pharmacies learned how to do their work through on-the-job training. Someone in the role of pharmacist's assistant was often a relative who came to work in the family business. The assistant assumed those responsibilities necessary to keep the business afloat while the pharmacist filled prescriptions and consulted with patients. Traditional corner druggists not only filled and dispensed prescriptions but also were the first-line health professionals with whom patients discussed their symptoms or their doctors' recommendations. Patients turned to pharmacists for advice and empathy.

As pharmacies evolved into divisions of big corporations, the owner-pharmacist became rarer. Nonpharmacist corporation owners viewed pharmacy as a revenue center that got customers into the store rather than as a patient-care provider. People working together in a pharmacy might not have known each other before the working relationship. Comprehensive on-the-job training of these individuals was a luxury requiring time no longer available to pharmacists in these settings. The need for documented proficiency of individuals performing technician's functions, however, did not go away. At the urging of pharmacy organizations, state boards of pharmacy developed regulations to guide in the training, role, and registration of technicians.

State Board Recognition of the Pharmacy Technician

State boards of pharmacy now set the requirements for being recognized as a pharmacy technician. Initially, experience counted as fulfilling the training aspect of registration or licensure (depending on the state). When states first started registering technicians, those who currently worked as technicians were grandfathered in—they simply applied for registration, and competency was implied. All the "grandfathers" have since been registered.

With technicians becoming more independently involved in filling orders and prescriptions, as well as in the associated clerical work and record keeping, standardized prerequisites are the norm. Formalized curriculum-based training best prepares technicians for these expanded responsibilities. Knowledge of basic medical terminology, diseases, and medications is fundamental in ensuring that they can ably record patient data and perform pharmacy distributive functions. Maintaining a professional demeanor and being able to converse with the variety of people encountered in a pharmacy practice should also be part of training.

When strangers meet, one way to assess the competency of one another is through standard measures. Education level is one accepted measure of a person's intellectual achievement. Certification examinations, as well as licensure examinations, are another way to ensure minimum competency. Qualifications for registration differ from state to state.

Most states require some defined minimum education experience. A high school diploma or GED is almost universally required. The number of hours of formal training as a technician varies from state to state. In some states, an associate's degree is required. In other states, a certificate attesting to the fact that the applicant has taken the prescribed number of class hours is sufficient. As the role of the technician expands, more and more states are also requiring certification by the Pharmacy Technician Certification Board (PTCB).

Certification

PTCB gives the certified pharmacy technician, or CPhT, examination three times a year. It tests the technician's competency for work in all aspects of pharmacy technology in the various practice sites. The examination consists of questions that evaluate calculations, filling prescriptions, maintaining profiles, and all the other technician functions that are part of the practice of pharmacy.

Aspiring technicians can prepare for the board and registration requirements for many states by enrolling in an ASHP-accredited pharmacy technology course. The curricula for these courses meet the minimum requirements set forth by ASHP. These courses include formal instruction in how the human body works, common diseases and conditions, and the medications used to treat them. They also provide

A national push for improving the safety of health care delivery is increasing the awareness of everyone on the provider side to the potential for errors.

exposure to and training in the specific responsibilities of a technician. Currently, courses must include a minimum of 600 hours of training time over a period of at least 15 weeks, although many run longer. Such intense training testifies to the level of commitment a person is willing to make for this type of career and allows for mastery of the material in a way that a short course does not.

State boards of pharmacy are increasingly requiring certification for registration or licensure. Registration is a formal sign up. Licensure carries a certain amount of responsibility for personal actions and usually requires some sort of test. In many states, the PTCB certification fulfills the test requirement and establishes a minimum level of competency. Also, with certification comes a continuing education requirement, which indicates that the technician is growing and continuing to keep abreast of the latest in pharmacy practice.

Medication Safety

A national push for improving the safety of health care delivery is increasing the awareness of everyone on the provider side to the potential for errors. The Institute for Safe Medication Practices (ISMP) is devoted to identifying errors, near misses, and potential errors. Through reports it receives from various institutions and practitioners, ISMP has brought situations from one arena to the attention of practitioners in other arenas so that errors are not repeated. ISMP has worked with regulators and the Food and Drug Administration (FDA) to establish guidelines and practices that promote safe medication use. One example is the FDA's recommendation to use so-called Tall Man lettering on bottles and containers of easily confused medications—for instance, hydrOXYzine and hydrALAZINE rather than hydroxyzine and hydralazine.

A collaborative effort between the Joint Commission accrediting body, stakeholders, and ISMP created the National Patient Safety Goals (NPSG). These goals are intended to inspire organizations to implement changes that improve patient safety. The 2009 goals that directly affect pharmaceutical care concern medication safety (NPSG 3) and medication reconciliation (NPSG 8).

Among other issues of medication safety, NPSG 3 identifies sound-alike and look-alike—or SALA—medications as an area for needed improvement. Sound-alike drugs are those with names that when spoken can be mistaken for other drugs. Names of look-alike drugs may be distinguishable when typed, but when they are written poorly, they can be read as other medications. Even with computerized order entry, some drug names are so similar that careless reading can lead to clicking on the wrong option. Table 13-1 gives some examples of SALA medications.

TABLE 13-1

Examples of Sound-Alike and Look-Alike Medications

Lantus	Lente
Humalog	Humulin
medroxyprednisolone	medroxyprogesterone
prochlorperazine	promethazine
Cortrosyn	cortisone
hydralazine	hydroxyzine
sertraline (Zoloft)	Seroquel (quetiapine)
clonidine	Klonopin (clonazepam)

Technicians can assist in reducing SALA errors. A common way that these errors are made is when it is assumed that a poorly written prescription or order is for a familiar product. Assumptions lead to errors. A great rule of thumb to go by is, "If you aren't absolutely sure, make the call—don't take the fall." Table 13-2 (page 188) gives some examples of drugs that can be confused if written carelessly.

Errors can be reduced by frequently reviewing medication names and becoming familiar with new products that may not be used every day in your setting. Another way to reduce errors is to ask the patient or read the chart to figure out why the doctor or prescriber wrote the prescription or order—that is, match indication or diagnosis with medication. Sometimes prescribers write the wrong medication because they too get confused with the sound-alike, look-alike names. Again, be aware that even with typewritten or computerized orders, errors can occur.

TABLE 13-2

Medications That Sound or Look Alike when Written Carelessly

Inderal	Imdur
hydromorphone (Dilaudid)	morphine
Depakote DR	Depakote ER
Zantac (ranitidine)	Xanax (alprazolam)
Celexa	Cerebryx
Wellbutrin SR	Wellbutrin XL
lamivudine	lamotrigine
doxorubicin	daunorubicin
paclitaxel (Taxol)	docetaxel (Taxotere)

The pharmacist is ultimately responsible for the correct medication getting to the patient, but an astute technician can ably assist in the process. You can point out orders that seem to have an excessive duration, such as an unusually long antibiotic course or a medication that seems to have a particularly high dose. Question orders that seem inconsistent with what you know about the patient or about the medication.

An astute technician is illustrated in the following example. A technician familiar with isosorbide noted that an order was written for isosorbide 100 mg taken three times a day. To get that dose, the patient would have to take at least two and a half of the 40 mg tablets or five of the 20 mg tablets. From experience, the technician determined that this dose was unusual. It turned out that the patient was really on isosorbide 10 mg taken three times a day—a decimal point error.

Errors in prescribing happen most often when a specialist such as a surgeon, ophthalmologist, or psychiatrist orders medication for a hospitalized patient that continues what the patient was taking at home. The regimen, perhaps initially prescribed by an internist, is frequently dictated by the patient from memory—or lack thereof. Because the specialist is often unfamiliar with typical doses or the use of the medication and relies only on information from the patient, an inappropriate dose may be prescribed. Such orders need to be checked carefully.

Bar Coding

Bar coding is another safety measure. The pharmaceutical societies, in conjunction with FDA and ISMP, have determined that bar coding prevents errors.

The premise for bar coding is that all elements in the system, including the patient, have a specific identity code. We're all familiar with bar codes on grocery items and the scanners used at checkout. In the health care system, each unit-dose medication has a bar code on the individual unit, as well as on the box it comes in. Some systems are sophisticated enough to show a picture of the medication so that a pharmacist can do a virtual inspection of it.

In bar-code systems, each patient has a unique bar code that appears on the patient's wristband or identification card. In the outpatient world, the patient's card is scanned at each point of service, and the medical record is pulled up. All services are linked to the bar code. Prescription orders, X-rays, procedures, and other orders are accessed via this unique code. Before an order is implemented, the card or wristband is scanned along with the order to ensure that the right service is going to the right patient. This concept has been referred to as the "smart card."

In the inpatient setting, the wristband and a bedside scanner are used. When administering a dose of medication to a patient at the bedside, the nurse scans the patient's wristband and the dose of medication. If the unit dose was not ordered for that patient or if it is the wrong dose or dosage form, such information is fed back to the nurse. At this final point for checking, the medication can be corrected before it is given to the patient. In addition, all personnel in the system are bar coded or given a unique numeric code so that each service can be traced to who delivered it to whom and at what time.

Bar coding of medication allows for electronic filling of cassettes as well as prescriptions. Many refill pharmacies already use a bar-code system to allow them to efficiently and quickly refill thousands of prescriptions with minimal personnel. Electronic filling of cassettes involves putting the medication in unit-dose fashion into a large filling machine. Of course, the only way that such a system can work well is with accurate coding and accurate labeling. An error in coding one medication could have major consequences in terms of the number of patients affected.

The premise for bar coding is that all elements in the system, including the patient, have a specific identity code.

Bar coding opens up new opportunities for technicians who like machinery. Stocking bar-code-based machines requires significant attention to detail. One small error in filling a machine can result in a significant number of subsequent errors because of the speed at which prescriptions or orders are filled. Besides ordering medications for the machines, technicians need to perform regular maintenance on them to keep them working efficiently. Systems have to be designed to remove expired medications from these devices in a timely manner. Methods need to be set up and responsibility given to change codes when a manufacturer's new product is exchanged for an old one or a new dosage form or strength comes on the market. Training for inputting data and maintenance of scanners and remote devices also needs to be developed.

The potential drawbacks of this system are significant. In a complete bar-code-based system, personnel may not be adequately trained for times when it breaks down. Will they be able to deliver medication quickly to patients if the whole system or parts of it shut down, as is apt to happen in an electronically based system? Will errors in filling the automated drug-storage compartments or entering information into a device's computer database be promptly detected before multiple patients have been delivered the wrong products? How will errors in information entered on patients be corrected if the "thinking" is done by computers?

Health Insurance and Universal Health Care

For decades, state and federal governments, insurance companies, businesses, health care providers, health care and other professional associations, the general public, and others have been wrestling with basic but thorny questions surrounding health insurance: What should be covered? Who should pay for it? Who should receive it? How should health care be delivered? How can costs be controlled? One of the few areas of agreement today is that the health care system is overburdened and sorely in need of overhauling.

One option that is being explored is universal health care, sometimes referred to as socialized medicine. This type of government insurance is available in a number of countries, including England, Sweden, and Canada. Proponents see it as a solution that gives everyone access to health care. Such health care systems do guarantee that all receive a minimum standard of health care. Opponents point to potential problems such as long waits, reduced overall quality of health care, and more restricted access to high-quality health care, especially for costlier services. In an article in the *British Medical Journal*,[2] a graph showed the decline of the number of people *waiting over six months* to be hospitalized. The same article points out the variation in health care between haves and have-nots despite universal health care. At this time, a health care system has not been created that is a perfect model for everyone.

Being aware of current events in your field increases the respect others have for you and your role in their health care.

These issues and others related to health care coverage are likely to continue to be debated for years to come. It's important to keep informed of developments—they will affect everyone working in health care.

Staying Current and Finding Out about Other Issues

Health care is on everyone's mind. When relatives and friends learn that you are a pharmacy technician, they may assume that you are also a medical care expert. In conversations about current health care events and articles in newspapers and magazines, you may be expected to clarify the issues.

It is a good idea to keep yourself informed about health care issues for several reasons. While you will not become an expert by reading a few articles, you will at least gain some knowledge. Being aware of current events in your field increases the respect others have for you and your role in their health care. In addition, it allows you to play a more active role on issues that may directly affect you. For instance, if you are working as a technician and are aware of a pending tech-check-tech bill, you could advocate for your position. There may be legislation limiting or expanding your role, changing the requirements for you to maintain your job, or altering how medication is dispensed. Although you may not always win, you can make a difference because by being informed, you can make contingency plans or orchestrate a compromise in your field.

Many opportunities exist in both the general media and professional literature for keeping informed. Radio or TV news programs in your area are among the easiest to access. Snippets gleaned from broadcasts on your way home from work can alert you to topics you might want or need to explore more extensively. Most local and national newspapers have articles on health topics. You can also catch up on health care issues by reading news magazines or even some of the women's or men's periodicals. Keep in mind that information from these sources introduces you to topics but may not be as accurate as information from reliable professional organizations. When news is reported in lay publications, remember to consult the original source documents as well.

In-depth information can be obtained from sources sponsored by health care professionals. These include professional journals published by organizations such as APhA, ASHP, the Massachusetts Medical Society, the American Diabetes Association, the American Neurological Association, and the Academy of Managed Care Pharmacy.

Professional seminars are another source of updates on the profession. Pharmacists often comment that they learn more in hallways than in classrooms—that is, casual conversations can be more informative than structured meetings and planned topics. Attending delegate sessions at national and state conferences informs you about political and legislative issues, and attending the educational seminars keeps you current on changes in disease management and new cures.

Finally, professionals can keep abreast of changes in the field by participating in home study programs or attending local seminars. Although some sponsored seminars may be biased, you can usually walk away with a lot of good information. Experience helps separate the reality from the hype.

Summary

Health care is an evolving field. Not long ago, health care meant treatment for a condition or illness. Today, it also includes prevention and maintenance. Medications change, and pharmaceutical discoveries are always occurring. The role of each player in the health care arena changes as the ways we deliver health care, pay for health care, and view health care change. Staying informed about changes in the field as they are evolving increases your success at dealing with change. Knowledge of changes can be obtained by reading lay and professional literature, listening to the news, and attending professional conferences and seminars.

ACTIVITIES

1. Read the health section of your local paper. What are some of the issues facing the practice of pharmacy today? How might they affect your career in 5 or 10 years?

2. How much do you think bar coding and electronic devices will help eliminate errors? What new problems will they bring?

3. Find an article on a health issue in a news magazine (e.g., *Time* or *Newsweek*). How does this issue affect pharmacy?

4. Imagine robotic pharmacies. Will there be a role for you in a self-serve setting?

5. Read a health-related article in the lay literature. Find its source article in the medical journal. How do these two articles compare with each other? What facts were left out of the lay article? Are they important?

References

1. Ambrose PJ, Saya FG, Lovett LT, et al. Evaluating the accuracy of technicians and pharmacists in checking unit dose medication cassettes. *Am J Health Syst Pharm*. 2002;59(12):1183–8.

2. Delamothe T. Universality, equity, and quality of care. *Br Med J*. 2008;336(7656):1278–81.

For More Information

Ambrose PJ, Saya FG, Lovett LT, et al. Evaluating the accuracy of technicians and pharmacists in checking unit dose medication cassettes. *Am J Health Syst Pharm*. 2002;59(12):1183–8.

American Journal of Health-System Pharmacy. Often publishes position statements analyzing issues, as well as studies supporting various viewpoints.

Coombes R. The NHS debate. *Br Med J*. 2008;337:a628.

Davies P. Flamingos? Nowt like that round here. *J R Soc Med.* 2008;101(5):219.

Delamothe T. Universality, equity, and quality of care. *Br Med J.* 2008;336(7656):1278–81.

Fontaine AL. Current requirements and emerging trends for labelling as a tool for communicating pharmacovigilance findings. *Drug Saf.* 2004;27(8):579–89.

Hadridge P, Pow R. What the NHS needs to improve: four behaviours to sort out the health system. *J R Soc Med.* 2008;101(1):7–11.

Journal of the American Pharmacists Association. A resource for current topics and trends in pharmacy practice, including regular updates on key issues concerning the field of pharmacy.

Medication bar coding and safety reporting to improve patient safety. *Public Health Rep.* 2003;118(3):275.

Muenzen PM, Corrigan MM, Smith MA, et al. Updating the pharmacy technician certification examination: a practice analysis study. *J Am Pharm Assoc.* 2006;46(1):e1–6.

Neuenschwander M, Cohen MR, Vaida AJ, et al. Practical guide to bar coding for patient medication safety. *Am J Health Syst Pharm.* 2003;60(8):768–79.

Bibliography

Arden P. *It's Not How Good You Are, It's How Good You Want to Be.* New York: Phaidon Press; 2003.

Benton, DA. *How to Think Like a CEO: The 22 Vital Traits You Need to Be the Person at the Top.* New York: Warner Books; 1999.

Berger BA. *Communication Skills for Pharmacists: Building Relationships, Improving Patient Care.* 3rd ed. Washington, DC: American Pharmacists Association; 2009.

Bittel LR, Newstrom JW. *What Every Supervisor Should Know.* 6th ed. New York: McGraw-Hill; 1992.

Covey SR, Merrill AR, Merrill RR. *First Things First.* New York: Simon & Schuster; 1994.

Covey SR. *The 7 Habits of Highly Effective People.* New York: Free Press; 2004.

Desselle SP, Zgarrick DP. *Pharmacy Management: Essentials for All Practice Settings.* 2nd ed. McGraw-Hill Medical; 2008.

Doyle M, Straus D. *How to Make Meetings Work.* New York: Jove Books; 1986.

Johnson S. *Who Moved My Cheese?* New York: G.P. Putnam's Sons; 1998.

Lawfer MA. *Why Customers Come Back: How to Create Lasting Customer Loyalty.* Franklin Lakes, NJ: Career Press; 2004.

Lundin SC, Paul H, Christensen J. *Fish! A Remarkable Way to Boost Morale and Improve Results.* New York: Hyperion; 2000.

McKain S. *What Customers Really Want: Bridging the Gap between What Your Company Offers and What Your Clients Crave.* Nashville, Tenn: Thomas Nelson; 2006.

Sigband NB. *Effective Communication for Pharmacists and Other Health Care Professionals.* Upland, Calif: Counterpoint Publications; 1995.

Viscott D. *Taking Care of Business: A Psychiatrist's Guide for True Success.* New York: William Morrow; 1985.

Index

Page numbers followed by t and f denote tables and figures, respectively.

A

Accessibility of private health information, 90
Accountability for private health information, 91
Acknowledgment of people's feelings, 41
Actions, personal, earning respect, 176
Active listening
    LAST approach to customer service, 39–41
    verbal communication, 7–8
Activities
    communication skills, 26
    customer service, 32–33
    diverse patient populations, 61
    Health Insurance Portability and
        Accountability Act (HIPAA), 92
    medication and inventory control systems, 127
    pharmacy practice issues, 193
    practice settings, role of the technician in,
        94, 106
    professionalism, 78
    staff management, 155
    team building, coaching, and mentoring, 175
    third-party payment issues, 117
    workflow management, 133, 137, 142, 143
Adults, addressing, 36–37
Advertising, 28
Agendas for meetings, 171, 171f
Ages of patients, 36–38
Alcohol consumption at office parties, 72–73
Alpha pagers, 74
American Pharmacists Association
    Code of Ethics, 83, 84–85f
    professional services, reimbursement for, 183
American Sign Language, 55
American Society of Health-System Pharmacists, 183
Americans with Disabilities Act, 55
Animals, working, 53
Answers to questions, 8–9, 8t
Assembly-line approach in retail pharmacy, 135
Assignment changes for staff, 157–159
Assisted living facilities, 101
Auto-attendants, 12
Automated dispensing machines, 138

B

Background checks for job applicants, 148
Bar coding, 189–190
Billing operations, workflow in, 140
Biological hoods, 98
Blind patients, 53–54
Body language
    body language to avoid, 10t
    cultural competence, 49–50
    nonverbal communication, 9–10
Bubble packaging, 101
Business letters, 22–23, 23t, 24f, 25f

C

Case managers for home health care pharmacy
    referral, 99
Cassette filling
    electronic, 189
    tech-check-tech accuracy, 180
    workflow management, 138
Cell phones, 73–74
Centralized stock, 133–134
Certification of pharmacy technicians, 185–186
Chemotherapy hoods, 98
Child-resistant caps and moisture resistance, 124
Children
    addressing, 37
    communication with, 36
Claims adjudication, online, 110, 116, 182
Class II drugs, 126–127
Cleanliness, personal, 64, 65, 66t
Clothing, professional, 64–65, 66t
Co-payments
    defined, 110
    tiered pricing plans, 111
Coaching staff members, 173–175
Codes of ethics, 83, 84–85f
Cold calling for personnel recruitment, 102
Communication
    cultural competence, 49–50
    management tool, 160–161
    pharmacy technology, success in, 94
    styles of, 8

Communication attributes
  compassion, 29
  encouragement, 31
  sincerity, 30–31
  sympathy and empathy, 30
Communication skills
  activities, 26
  communication, forms of, 5–6
  nonverbal communication, 9–10, 10t
  summary, 23
  verbal communication: in person, 7–9, 8t
  verbal communication: telephone, 10–13, 13–14t
  written communication
    e-mail, 14–19, 15f, 16f, 17f, 18f, 19–20t
    intradepartmental notes, 20–21, 21t
    letters, 22–23, 23t, 24f, 25f
    memos, 22
Community pharmacy practice, 94–95
Compassion
  cultural competence, 48
  expressing, 29
Competency assessment
  new staff, 153–154
  periodic, 154
Complementary and alternative medicine, 51
Compounding of sterile products, 97–98
Compounding pharmacies, 95–96
Computer systems
  accountability for private health information, 91
  interface systems for inventory ordering, 121
Computerized physician order entry (CPOE), 180
Conceptual managers, 160
Confidentiality
  discipline of staff, 156
  professionalism, 71
Conflict in the workplace, 163–164
Consistency in management, 162–163
Continuity of care, 89
Contracts with employees, 159
Controlled substances, 126–127
Controlling managers, 160
Costs, share of, paid by patients, 109–111
CPOE (computerized physician order entry), 180
Credit for returns of inventory, 124
Cross-training, 131–132
Cultures
  conflicts, resolving, 59–60
  cultural competence, 48–49
  influences on health care, 47–48, 47t
  learning about, 58–59
Customer service
  activity, 32–33
  attributes for professional communication, 29–31

business reception, 28–29
customers and patients, attracting and keeping, 27–28
customers of different ages, 36–38
difficult patients, 38–39
LAST approach, 39–44
summary, 44
winning in business, 31, 33–36
Customers
  greeting, 70
  identifying, 67–68, 68t
  interacting with, 68–69, 69t

D
DEA (U.S. Drug Enforcement Administration), 126–127
DEA 222 form, 126–127
DEA numbers, 126
Deaf patients, 54–56
Decentralized stock, 133–134
Decision-making, cultural differences in, 50, 52
Deductibles, 109–110
Demeanor, personal, 68
Diagnoses, on treatment authorization requests, 114, 115f
Diagnosis-related groups (DRGs)
  private health information, 90
  reimbursement, 182
Difficult patients, dealing with, 38–39
Discharge planners for home health care pharmacy referral, 99
Discipline, administering to staff, 156, 157f
Disclosure rule, 83
Dispensing pharmacies, 96–97
Diverse patient populations
  activities, 61
  cultural competence, 48–49
  cultural conflicts, resolving, 59–60
  cultural differences in pharmacy situations, 50–51
  cultural influences on health care, 47–48, 47t
  incorporating knowledge into practice, 51–52
  language and communication styles, 49–50
  other cultures, learning about, 58–59
  patients with physical challenges, 52–56, 56t
  political correctness and language choices, 56–57
  religion, 57–58
  summary, 60–61
Documentation
  investigational drug trials, 103, 104
  staff management, 160
  third-party payers, submitting to, 110
"Donut hole" in Medicare Part D policies, 110

Double-blind studies, 104
Drug information sites, responsibilities in, 104–105
Durable medical equipment sales, 99
Durable power of attorney, 52

E

E-mail
  advantages and disadvantages, 14–15
  brief and direct, 15f, 16
  do's and don'ts, 19–20t
  emotional responses, 15, 16–17, 16f
  mass distributions, 17–19, 17f, 18f
  reprimands, 18–19, 18f
Elderly customers
  communicating with, 37–38
  cultural differences, 50
  cultural norms, 48
Electronic cassette filling, 189
Emotional e-mail, 15, 16–17, 16f
Empathy
  cultural competence, 48
  expressing, 30
  professionalism, 71
Encouragement
  cultural competence, 48
  expressing, 31
Engaging another person, in verbal
      communication, 7
Errors
  prescriptions, in, 188
  sound-alike and look-alike medications, 187,
      187t
  taking responsibility for, 74–76
  written prescriptions, 187–188, 188t
Errors in judgment, 75–76
Errors of omission, 76
Ethics
  business, effect on, 82–83
  business practices, 79–82
  codes of, 83, 84–85f
  described, 78–79
Expiration dates, 124
Eye contact
  cultural competence, 49–50
  nonverbal communication, 10

F

Family members as sign-language interpreters, 56
FDA. See U.S. Food and Drug Administration (FDA)
Feedback
  management tool, 160–161
  negative, 155
  performance, on, 154–155
  verbal communication, 9

Financial investment in inventory, 120
Firing staff, 156
Five rights of medication, 75
Flexibility in workflow, 131–132
Floor stock inspections, 98
Formal performance reviews, 156
Formularies, 111–112

G

Gestures, 49–50
Golden Rule, 82
Grammar, 9
Guide dogs, 53

H

Hands, appearance of, 65–66
Healing animals, 53
Health care issues
  cultural variations, 47t
  staying current in, 191–192
Health insurance companies
  health insurance, issues in, 190–191
  private health information, 90
  third-party payment issues, 109
Health Insurance Portability and Accountability
      Act (HIPAA)
  accessibility of information, 90
  accountability, 91
  activity, 92
  health information, protection of, 87–88
  "need to know" issues, 90
  patient confidentiality, 71
  portability of information, 89
  private health information, explained, 87
  summary, 91
Hearing-impaired patients, 54–56
HIPAA. See Health Insurance Portability and
      Accountability Act (HIPAA)
Hiring
  interviewing, 146–148, 147t
  reasons for, 146
  references for applicants, 148–151, 149f, 150f,
      152f
Hispanic cultures, 49
Hold, placing caller on, 11
Home health care pharmacies, 98–100
Hospital pharmacies
  satellite and dispensing pharmacies, 96–97
  sterile compounding, 97–98
  workflow management, 137–139
Human resources department, 159–160

I

Informed consent for investigational drug trials, 103
Infusion centers, 102
Institute for Safe Medication Practices, 186
Interviewing job applicants, 146–148, 147t
Intradepartmental notes, 20–21, 21t
Intravenous admixtures, compounding, 97
Inventory
    appropriate levels, deciding, 120–121
    centralized and decentralized, 133–134
    control systems, 119, 119t
    controlled substances, 126–127
    hospital settings, 98
    ordering, 121–122
    stock rotation and regular maintenance, 124
Investigational drug trials, pharmacies associated
    with, 103–104

J

Joint Commission
    expiration dates, checking, 124
    medication safety, 186
Justifications, on treatment authorization
    requests, 114, 115f

L

Lab coats, 66
Language
    cultural competence, 49–50
    cultural or physical differences, 57
    verbal communication, 9
Large orders in retail pharmacy, 136–137
LAST approach to customer service, 39–44
Leadership versus management, 176
Learned skills for pharmacy technology, 93
Legal issues, human resources, 159
Letters
    business letters, 22–23, 23t, 24f, 25f
    recommendation letters for job applicants,
        148–151, 149f, 150f, 152f
    warning letters to staff, 156, 157f
Licensure of pharmacy technicians, 186
Life-cycle events
    cultural influences on, 47t, 48
    rituals, cultural differences in, 49
Light sensitivity of medications, 123
Lip reading by patients, 55
Listening
    active listening, 7–8, 39–41
    LAST approach to customer service, 39–41
    professionalism, 71
    sincerity, expressing, 30

Long-term care facilities
    role of pharmacy technician, 101
    workflow management, 137–139

M

Mail-order pharmacies, 100–101
Management. *See also* Staff management;
        Workflow management
    versus leadership, 176
    styles, 160–161
Manners
    meetings, for, 77
    workplace, 73
Mass-distribution e-mail, 17–19, 17f, 18f
Mediator, manager as, in workplace conflicts,
        164–165
Medicaid as third-party payer, 109
Medicare
    medication therapy management, 180, 183
    third-party payment issues, 109
Medicare Part D, 110
Medication and inventory control systems
    activities, 127
    appropriate stock levels, 120–121
    inventory control, elements of, 119, 119t
    narcotics and other controlled substances,
        126–127
    orders, checking in, 122
    returns and recalls, 124–126
    routine ordering, 121–122
    stock rotation and regular maintenance, 124
    storage requirements, 122–124, 123f
    summary, 127
Medication therapy management (MTM),
        180–181, 183
Medications
    formularies, in, 111–112
    restricted, in formularies, 112
    safety issues, 186–188, 187t, 188t
    shortages, 121
Meetings
    professionalism, 77
    strategies for conducting, 172
    team building, 171–173, 171f
Memos, 22
Mentoring staff, 173–175
Message machines, 12
Minutes of meetings, 172–173
Misunderstandings
    e-mail, 15
    verbal communication, 9
Moisture, medication sensitivity to, 123, 124
Monitoring visits for sponsored studies, 104
MTM (medication therapy management),
        180–181, 183

N

Nails, appearance of, 65–66
Narcotics, control of, 126–127
National Drug Code (NDC) numbers, 116
National Patient Safety Goals, 186–187
Native American cultures, 49
"Need to know" in private health information, 90
Negative feedback, 155
Nonjudgmental actions, 51
Nonverbal communication, 9–10, 10t

O

Office parties, 72–73
Offices, workflow management in, 140
Online claims adjudication, 110, 116, 182
Open-door policy for management, 175
Opposite sex, cultural differences regarding, 50
Orders
    changes in, 138–139
    checking in, 122
    routine, 121–122
Oversystematizing workflow management,
    130–132

P

Package inserts, 122–123, 123f
Pagers, 74
Paperwork. *See* Documentation
Par-level system of inventory ordering, 121
Patient demands, cultural sensitivity to, 51
Perception by customers, 33
Performance
    feedback on, 154–155
    formal reviews, 156
Periodic feedback on performance, 155
Personal space, 9
Personality traits for pharmacy technicians, 94
Personnel recruitment functions, 101–102
Pharmacy benefits manager companies, 105
Pharmacy practice issues
    activities, 193
    bar coding, 189–190
    health insurance and universal health care,
        190–191
    medication safety, 186–188, 187t, 188t
    medication therapy management, 180–181
    reimbursement, 181–183
    staying current, 191–192
    summary, 192–193
    tech-check-tech, 179–180
    technician education and certification,
        183–186
Pharmacy profession, evolution of, 1–2

Pharmacy technician education and certification
    certification, 185–186
    historical perspective, 183–184
    state board recognition of the pharmacy
        technician, 184–185
Pharmacy technicians
    increased need for, 2
    management issues, familiarity with, 2–3
Physical challenges
    guidelines for dealing with patients with
        physical disabilities, 56t
    patients with, 52–56
Physical layout
    impediments to workflow, 132–133
    workflow management, 139–140, 140t
Physical skills for pharmacy technology, 93
Planned work in retail pharmacy, 136
Political correctness, 56–57
Portability of health information, 89
Positioning of information as communication
    method, 6
Positive pressure rooms for sterile compounding, 97
Posture
    nonverbal communication, 9–10
    professionalism, 68
Practice settings, role of the technician in
    activities, 94, 106
    community pharmacy practice, 94–95
    compounding pharmacies, 95–96
    drug information sites, 104–105
    home health care pharmacies, 98–100
    hospital settings, 96–98
    infusion centers, 102
    long-term care, 101
    mail-order pharmacies, 100–101
    personnel recruitment functions, 101–102
    pharmacies associated with investigational
        drug trials, 103–104
    pharmacy benefits manager companies, 105
    satellite and dispensing pharmacies, 96–97
    skills needed for pharmacy technology, 93–94
    sterile compounding, 97–98
    summary, 106
Prescriptions, multiple, in retail pharmacy, 136–137
Prioritizing
    general rules for, 142–143
    workflow strategy, 141–142
Private health information
    cultural differences in access to, 50–51, 52
    explained, 87
    protection of, 87–88
Problems
    difficult questions by patients, 72
    LAST approach to customer service, 41–43
    workflow delays, 139

Professional journals, 192
Professional pharmacist services, reimbursement for, 181, 182–183
Professional practice, cultural competence in, 51–52
Professional seminars, 192
Professionalism and ethics in the workplace
  activities, 78
  cell phones and pagers, 73–74
  customers, greeting, 70
  customers, identifying and interacting with, 67–69, 68t, 69t
  difficult questions, answering, 71–72
  empathy and sympathy, 71
  ethics, 78–83, 84–85f
  manners in the workplace, 73
  meetings, 77
  office parties, 72–73
  patient confidentiality, 71
  professional appearance, 63–66, 66t
  professionalism, elements of, 69t
  responsibility, taking, 74–76
  summary, 85
  timeliness, 76
Public relations in home health care pharmacies, 99

Q
Questions
  answers as communication style, 8–9, 8t
  difficult questions by patients, 71–72
  interviewing job applicants, 147, 147t

R
Recalls of inventory, 125–126
Reception of clients, 28–29
References/recommendation letters for job applicants, 148–151, 149f, 150f, 152f
Registration of pharmacy technicians, 186
Reimbursement issues, 181–183
Relationships with customers, 28
Religion, accommodation for, 57–58
"Reply all" feature of e-mail, 17
Reprimands to groups in e-mail, 18–19, 18f
Respect
  customer service, 28
  generating, 175–176
  teamwork, 169
  work environment, in, 163
Responsibility, taking, 74–76
Retail pharmacy
  role of pharmacy technician in, 94–95
  workflow management, 135–137
Returns of inventory, 124–125

Rotation of assignments, 131–132
Rotation of stock, 124

S
Safety issues, 186–188, 187t, 188t
Sales positions at home health care pharmacies, 99
Satellite pharmacies, 96–97
Seated positions as nonverbal communication, 9–10
Self-awareness as management asset, 160
Sign-language interpreters, 55–56
Sincerity, expressing, 30–31
Single-blind studies, 104
Skilled nursing facilities, 101
Skills. See also Communication skills
  learned, for pharmacy technology, 93
  periodic assessment of, 154
  physical, 93
  staff development, 157–159
"Smart cards," 189
Smiling when using the telephone, 11
Social issues with cultural variations, 47t
Sound-alike and look-alike medications, 187–188, 187t, 188t
Space management for workflow, 139–140, 140t
Sponsored studies, 104
Staff management
  activity, 163
  assessment of staff, 145–146
  assignment changes and skill development, 157–159
  feedback on performance, 154–155
  formal performance reviews, 156
  hiring, 146–151, 147t, 149f, 150f, 152f
  human resources department, 159–160
  internal conflict prevention and management, 163–166
  interviewing to hire, 146–148, 147t
  management styles, 160–161
  negative feedback, giving, 155
  new staff, testing competency of, 153–154
  new staff, training, 151, 153–154
  periodic skill assessment, 154
  pleasant work environment, maintaining, 162–163
  productive staff, managing, 161
  references for applicants, 148–151, 149f, 150f, 152f
  summary, 166–167
  unpleasant news, delivering, 156, 157f
Standing position as nonverbal communication, 9
State boards of pharmacy, 184–185
Steps, saving, 139–140, 140t
Sterile compounding, 97–98

Stock. *See* Inventory
Storage requirements for medications, 122–124, 123f
"Sunshine rule," 83
Support groups, speaking to, 99
Surroundings, awareness of, 69
Sympathy
cultural competence, 48
expressing, 30
professionalism, 71

T

Tall Man lettering, 186
Tangible services, reimbursement for, 181
Tasks, order of, to manage workflow, 134–134
Team approach in retail pharmacy, 135
Team building, coaching, and mentoring
activity, 175
coaching and mentoring, 173–175
leadership versus management, 176
meetings, 171–173, 171f
respect, generating upward, 175–176
summary, 177
teamwork, 169–170
Teamwork
barriers to, 170
building, 169, 170
Tech-check-tech, 179–180
Technology for mail-order pharmacies, 100–101
Telecommunications devices for the deaf (TDD), 55–56
Telephone use
tips for successful, 13–14t
verbal communication, 10–13
Temperature for medication storage, 122, 123, 123f
Thank you, saying
e-mail to colleagues, 18–19, 18f
LAST approach to customer service, 43–44
letters, 24f
Third-party payment issues
activities, 117
claims adjudication, 116
costs, share of paid by patients, 109–111
formularies, 111–112
reimbursement issues, 182
sources of payment, 109
summary, 116
treatment authorization requests, 112–114, 113f, 115f
Tiered pricing plans for formularies, 111
Timeliness, 76
Total parenteral nutrition, compounding, 97

Treatment authorization requests
pharmacy benefits manager companies, 105
third-party payers, 112–114, 113f, 115f
Trips, planning in managing workflow, 139
Turnover of inventory, 120

U

Unit-dose system, 96–97
United States Pharmacopeia (USP) 797 guidelines, 95, 97
Universal health care, 190–191
Unplanned work in retail pharmacy, 136
U.S. Drug Enforcement Administration (DEA), 126–127
U.S. Food and Drug Administration (FDA)
investigational drug trials, pharmacies associated with, 103, 104
medication safety, 186
recalls of drugs, 124

V

Verbal communication
advantages of, 5
in person, 7–9, 8t
telephone, 10–13, 13–14t
uses for, 6
Verbal shorthand, 8–9
Visually impaired patients, 53–54

W

Warning letters to staff, 156, 157f
Winning in business, 31, 33–36
Word use. *See* Language
Work environment, pleasant, maintaining, 162–163
Workflow management
activities, 133, 137, 142, 143
centralized and decentralized stock, 133–134
good workflow, designing, 129, 129t
hospital and long-term care issues, 137–139
large orders, 136–137
oversystematizing, 130–132
physical impediments to maximizing workflow, 132–133
physical layout, 139–140, 140t
planned and unplanned work, 136
prioritizing, 141–143
problems delaying workflow, 139
retail settings, issues in, 135–137
summary, 143
tasks, order of, 134–135
trips, planning, 139
Working animals, 53

Written communication
        advantages of, 5–6
        e-mail, 14–19, 15f, 16f, 17f, 18f, 19–20t
        hearing-impaired patients, 54–55
        intradepartmental notes, 20–21, 21t
        letters, 22–23, 23t, 24f, 25f
        memos, 22
        uses for, 6

Y
Younger people, cultural norms of, 48